Pediatric Emergency Radiology

T0202358

What Do I Do Now?: Emergency Medicine

SERIES EDITOR-IN-CHIEF

Catherine A. Marco, MD, FACEP
Professor, Emergency Medicine & Surgery
Wright State University Boonshoft School of Medicine
Dayton, Ohio

Pediatric Emergency Radiology

Edited by
Ann Dietrich

Associate Editor
Gayathri Sreedher

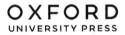

OXFORD
UNIVERSITY PRESS

Oxford University Press is a department of the University of Oxford. It furthers
the University's objective of excellence in research, scholarship, and education
by publishing worldwide. Oxford is a registered trade mark of Oxford University
Press in the UK and certain other countries.

Published in the United States of America by Oxford University Press
198 Madison Avenue, New York, NY 10016, United States of America.

Library of Congress Cataloging-in-Publication Data
Names: Dietrich, Ann M., editor. | Sreedher, Gayathri, editor.
Title: Pediatric emergency radiology / editor, Ann Dietrich; associate editor, Gayathri Sreedher.
Description: New York, NY : Oxford University Press, [2023] |
Includes bibliographical references and index.
Identifiers: LCCN 2022040656 (print) | LCCN 2022040657 (ebook) |
ISBN 9780197628553 (paperback) | ISBN 9780197628577 (epub) |
ISBN 9780197628584 (online)
Subjects: MESH: Emergencies | Child | Infant | Radiology |
Pediatric Emergency Medicine | Case Reports
Classification: LCC RJ370 (print) | LCC RJ370 (ebook) | NLM WS 205 |
DDC 618.92/0025—dc23/eng/20230103
LC record available at https://lccn.loc.gov/2022040656
LC ebook record available at https://lccn.loc.gov/2022040657

DOI: 10.1093/med/9780197628553.001.0001

9 8 7 6 5 4 3 2 1

Printed by Marquis, Canada

Contents

Contributors

Peter Assaad, MD, MPH, MBA
Lurie Children's Hospital
Chicago, IL, USA

Isabel A. Barata, MS, MD, MBA
Professor of Pediatrics and
  Emergency Medicine
Department of Emergency
  Medicine
Donald and Barbara Zucker
  School of Medicine at
  Hofstra/Northwell
Ozone Park, NY, USA

Berkeley Bennett, MD, MS
Attending Physician
Department of Emergency
Nationwide Children's Hospital,
  The Ohio State University
Columbus, OH, USA

Beth Bubolz, MD
Assistant Professor
Department of Pediatrics
The Ohio State University College
  of Medicine
Lewis Center, OH, USA

Francesca M. Bullaro, MD
Associate Trauma Medical Director,
  Assistant Professor
Pediatric Emergency Medicine
Cohen Children's Medical Center
  Northwell Health
Garden City, NY, USA

Zachary Burroughs, MD
Clinical Assistant Professor
Emergency Medicine, Division of
  Pediatric Emergency Medicine
Prisma Health Upstate
Greenville, SC, USA

Ailish Coblentz, MBBS, FRCPC
Assistant Professor and Paediatric
  Radiologist
Department of Diagnostic Imaging
The Hospital for Sick Children,
  University of Toronto
Toronto, ON, CA

Thomas P. Conway, DO
Physician Fellow
Department of Pediatric
  Emergency Medicine
Cohen Children's Medical Center
Astoria, NY, USA

Kristol Das, MD
Fellow
Department of Pediatric
  Emergency Medicine
Nationwide Children's Hospital
Columbus, OH, USA

Ann Dietrich, MD
Professor of Pediatrics and Emergency
  Medicine, University of South
  Carolina College of Medicine
Department of Emergency Medicine
Division Chief Pediatric
  Emergency Medicine, PRISMA
Greenville, SC, USA

Meika Eby, MD, FAAP
Department of Pediatrics
Nationwide Children's
    Hospital, The Ohio State
    University
Columbus, OH, USA

David Fernandez, MD
Chief Resident-Education
Department of Emergency Medicine
Northwell: Northshore-LIJ
    Hospital
Astoria, NY, USA

David Foster, MD, MS
Assistant Professor
Departments of Emergency
    Medicine and Pediatrics
Associate Director EM Residency
    Program, Northwell Health,
    Zucker School of Medicine
Manhasset, NY, USA

**Shankar Srinivas Ganapathy,
    MBBS, MD**
Pediatric Radiologist, Associate
    Professor of Radiology
    at NEOMED
Department of Radiology
Akron Children's Hospital
Akron, OH, USA

Robert L. Gates, MD
Professor
Department of Surgery
University of South Carolina
    School of Medicine—Greenville
Greenville, SC, USA

Rachelle Goldfisher, MD
Associate Chief
Department of Pediatric
    Radiology
Northwell Health
Queens, NY, USA

Sophia Gorgens, MD
Resident
Department of Emergency
    Medicine
Zucker-Northwell North Shore/
    Long Island Jewish
Manhasset, NY, USA

Cory Gotowka, DO, MS
Pediatric Hospitalist
UPMC Hamot
Erie, PA

Michelle Greene, DO
Assistant Professor
Division of Emergency Medicine,
    Department of Pediatrics
The Ohio State University
    College of Medicine, and
    Nationwide Children's
    Hospital, Columbus, OH
Columbus, OH, USA

Yamini Jadcherla, MD
Pediatric Emergency
    Medicine Fellow
Department of Pediatric
    Emergency Medicine
Nationwide Children's Hospital
Galena, OH, USA

Dana Kaplan, MD
Director of Child Abuse and Neglect
Department of Pediatrics
Staten Island University Hospital
Marlboro, NJ, USA

Jane S. Kim, MD
Assistant Professor of Pediatrics and
 Radiology
Division of Diagnostic Imaging
 and Radiology
Children's National Hospital
Kensington, MD, USA

George C. Koberlein, MD
Associate Professor
Department of Radiology
Atrium Health at Wake Forest Baptist
Winston-Salem, NC, USA

Rajesh Krishnamurthy, MD
Director, Cardiothoracic Imaging
Department of Radiology
Nationwide Children's Hospital
Dublin, OH, USA

Brooke Lampl, DO, FAOCR
Staff Radiologist/Clinical Assistant
 Professor of Radiology
Department of Diagnostic Radiology
Cleveland Clinic
Pepper Pike, OH, USA

William Mak, DO
Attending Physician
Department of Pediatrics
Cohen Children's Medical Center
Flushing, NY, USA

Deanna Margius, MD
Resident
Department of Emergency Medicine
Hofstra Northwell NS-LIJ
Manhasset, NY, USA

Lauren May, MD
Nemours Children's Hospital,
 Delaware, Wilmington, DE
Clinical Assistant Professor
Department of Radiology and
 Pediatrics
Sidney Kimmel School of Medicine
 Thomas Jefferson University
Philadelphia, PA

Aaron McAllister, MS, MD
Assistant Professor
Department of Radiology
Nationwide Children's Hospital
Columbus, OH, USA

Melissa A. McGuire, MD
Assistant Professor and Associate
 Program Director of Northwell
 Health CCMC Pediatric
 Emergency Medicine Fellowship
Department of Emergency Medicine
Northwell Health, Cohen
 Children's Medical Center and
 North Shore University Hospital
Massapequa Park, NY, USA

McKenzie Montana, DO
Resident Physician
Department of Pediatrics
Prisma Health-Upstate
Greenville, SC, USA

Waroot S. Nimjareansuk, DO
Assistant Professor
Department of Orthopaedics and
Sports Medicine
University of Florida
Minneola, FL, USA

Nkeiruka Orajiaka, MBBS, MPH
Pediatrician, Assistant Professor
Department of Emergency
Medicine
Nationwide Children's Hospital,
The Ohio State University
Columbus, OH, USA

Gina Pizzitola, MD, MS
Pediatric Emergency
Medicine Fellow
Department of Pediatric
Emergency Medicine
Cohen Children's Medical Center,
Northwell Health
Glen Oaks, NY, USA

Ajay K. Puri, MD
Fellow, Montefiore Medical
Center
Critical Care Medicine
North Shore University
Hospital
Forest Hills, NY, USA

Mantosh S. Rattan, MD
Staff Radiologist
Department of Radiology
Cleveland Clinic Foundation
Cincinnati, OH, USA

Maegan S. Reynolds, MD
Assistant Professor of Emergency
Medicine and Pediatrics
Department of Emergency
Medicine The Ohio State
University and Division of
Pediatric Emergency
Medicine Nationwide Children's
Fracture
Columbus, OH, USA

Esther Ro, MD
Instructor of Radiology
Department of Radiology
Northwestern University Feinberg
School of Medicine
Wilmette, IL, USA

Joshua Rocker, MD
Associate Professor and
Division Chief
Department of Pediatric
Emergency Medicine
Cohen Children's Medical Center
New Hyde Park, NY, USA

Emily Rose, MD
Associate Professor of Clinical
Emergency Medicine
(Educational Scholar)
Department of Emergency
Medicine
Keck School of Medicine of
the University of Southern
California
Arcadia, CA, USA

Bindu N. Setty, MD
Clinical Associate Professor
Department of Radiology
Boston University
Lexington, MA, USA

Summit Shah, MD, MPH
Pediatric Radiologist
Department of Radiology
Nationwide Children's
    Hospital
Columbus, OH, USA

Narendra Shet, MD
Associate Professor and Director
    of Body MR
Division of Diagnostic Imaging
    and Radiology
Children's National Hospital
Ellicott City, MD, USA

Michael Sperandeo, MD
Attending Physician
Department of Emergency
    Medicine
Long Island Jewish Medical
    Center
Long Beach, NY, USA

Gayathri Sreedher, MBBS, MD
Staff Pediatric Radiologist
Department of Radiology
Akron Children's Hospital
Akron, OH, USA

Michael Stoner, MD
Associate Professor and
    Section Chief
Department of Pediatrics/Division
    of Emergency Medicine
The Ohio State University College
    of Medicine and Nationwide
    Children's Hospital
Canal Winchester, OH, USA

David Teng, MD
Assistant Professor
Department of Pediatrics, Division
    of Emergency Medicine
Cohen Children's Medical
    Center—Northwell Health
Dix Hills, NY, USA

Anna Thomas, MD
Clinical Associate Professor
Department of Radiology
Children's Hospital of Los
    Angeles, USC Keck School of
    Medicine
Redlands, CA, USA

Linda Vachon, MD
Associate Professor of Clinical
    Radiology
Department of Radiology
University of Southern California,
    Keck School of Medicine
Manhattan Beach, CA, USA

Esben Vogelius, MD
Radiologist
Department of Radiology
Cleveland Clinic
Moreland Hills, OH, USA

Kristy Williamson, MD
Associate Chief
 Department of Pediatric Emergency
Cohen Children's Medical Center
Garden City, NY, USA

Madeline Zito, DO, FAAP
Department of Pediatrics
Maimonides Children's Hospital
Brooklyn, NY, USA

1   Walking and Wheezing

Rajesh Krishnamurthy and Beth Bubolz

Case Study

A 16-year-old male with no past medical history and a recent viral infection (not COVID) presents with 1 month of cough, shortness of breath, and wheezing with walking. He must frequently stop and rest when walking outside, has trouble going up the stairs, and has stopped participating in sports. He also has decreased appetite with associated nausea, vomiting, and abdominal pain off and on for a few weeks.

He was seen by his pediatrician 2 weeks ago for vague abdominal pain, nausea and diarrhea and was diagnosed with gastroenteritis and was discharged with ondansetron. Vital signs and physical examination at that visit were normal.

His cough is currently dry. Vital signs are: blood pressure 100/67mmHg; pulse 106 beats per minute; temperature 97.8°F (36.6°C); respiratory rate 20 breaths per minute; weight 62.4 kg; oxygen saturation (SpO2) 93%. He is well-appearing. Lungs are clear and his heart sounds are normal, with no murmur. Abdominal exam reveals no pain or masses, with a normal sized liver.

While completing the exam, he vomits, becomes pale, diaphoretic, and tachypneic.

What do you do now?

DISCUSSION

An adolescent with cough, shortness of breath, and wheezing has a differential that includes asthma, pneumothorax, pneumonia, achalasia, myocarditis, and congestive heart failure (HF).

Patients with asthma, a chronic inflammatory disease of the airways, typically have recurrent episodes of airflow obstruction resulting from edema, bronchospasm, and increased mucus production in the airways. Children frequently have associated seasonal allergies (allergic rhinitis) and eczema (atopic dermatitis), with these three conditions forming what is known as the atopic triad. This patient does not have a history of allergic diseases or wheezing and on physical exam is not currently wheezing.

Children have an increased risk of pneumothorax with a previous history of an emphysematous bleb, asthma (10%), and tobacco use (4%). An underlying congenital anomaly might also serve as a predisposing factor, particularly in a younger child. Young males with Marfan syndrome, the most common inherited disorder of connective tissue, are also more likely to have a spontaneous pneumothorax. Clinically, children usually present with the acute onset of pain at rest or during physical activity and, depending on the size of the pneumothorax, might have dyspnea and cough. Physical exam findings may reveal differences in air entry to the lungs; however, with a small pneumothorax, unequal breath sounds, hyperresonance with percussion, and asymmetric wall movements might be subtle or not yet present. This child does not have risk factors or findings associated with a pneumothorax.

Achalasia is a rare esophageal neurodegenerative disorder that may occur in the pediatric population. Achalasia may be associated with other conditions including Trisomy 21, congenital hypoventilation syndrome, glucocorticoid insufficiency, eosinophilic esophagitis, familial dysautonomia, Chagas' disease, and achalasia, alacrima, and adrenocorticotropic hormone (ACTH) insensitivity (AAA) syndrome. Children afflicted with achalasia usually present with progressive dysphagia, vomiting, and weight loss. Recurrent pneumonia, nocturnal cough, aspiration, hoarseness, and feeding difficulties may occur in younger children. Although this patient has vomiting, he does not have progressive dysphagia, making this diagnosis unlikely.

Usually, acute myocarditis presents with preceding viral symptoms (about two-thirds of patients), HF symptoms, and a poorly functioning ventricle with or without dilation. Fulminant myocarditis may present with tachyarrhythmias and significant cardiac dysfunction. A history of a preceding viral prodrome is commonly present (two-thirds of patients); ventricular and atrial arrhythmias are also common (about 45%). Sudden cardiac death may also be a presentation of myocarditis. Complications of myocarditis may include a dilated cardiomyopathy or a pericardial effusion.

The clinicians for this patient started with a chest radiograph. The initial chest radiographic identified small pleural effusions and interlobular septal thickening, which were suggestive of interstitial pulmonary edema (see Figures 1.1a and 1.1b). Findings become more apparent when compared with a normal 16-year-old's chest radiographs (Figures 1.2a and 1.2b). Because of the patient's vomiting, an abdominal film was also obtained, which demonstrated significant cardiomegaly (see Figure 1.1c), thus leading to the diagnosis of dilated cardiomyopathy and/or pericardial effusion. On the chest radiograph, the reduced lung volumes and elevated hemidiaphragms masked the cardiomegaly, which was more apparent on the better penetrated abdominal radiograph.

Careful attention to the heart, mediastinum, airway, lungs, pleura, bones, and soft tissues is essential to accurately diagnose the cause of chest pain. A screening chest film for patients with chest pain has low sensitivity for structural cardiovascular lesions, such as myocarditis, dissection, or pulmonary infarction, but is helpful in the acute setting to diagnose complications of underlying cardiovascular conditions, such as HF, mediastinal hematoma, or pulmonary infarction. It is also helpful to exclude noncardiac causes of chest pain, including pneumonia, pneumothorax, rib fracture, or an aspirated foreign body (see normal chest radiograph, Figures 1.2a and 1.2b).

In addition, the physician ordered an electrocardiogram (ECG). An ECG with a chest radiograph is a great screening tool set for cardiomyopathy of any type. ECGs are particularly valuable in patients who present with symptoms that may be suspicious for cardiac involvement and include dyspnea, fatigue, shortness of breath, tachypnea, unexplained tachycardia, murmur, gallop, rub, vague abdominal pain, etc.

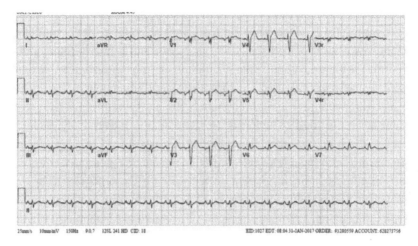

ECG demonstrates sinus tachycardia, low voltage, borderline long QT interval, and mild conduction delay in V1.

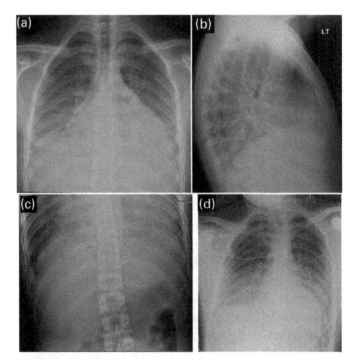

FIGURES 1.1a, 1.1b, 1.1c, AND 1.1d. (a, b) PA and lateral views of the chest demonstrating low lung volumes, pulmonary vascular congestion, interstitial opacities in the lung bases, and bilateral trace pleural fluid; (c) the abdominal radiograph is better penetrated than the chest radiograph, and shows an enlarged cardiac silhouette; and (d) post-procedure chest radiograph showing decreased size of the cardiac silhouette after drainage of the pericardial effusion.

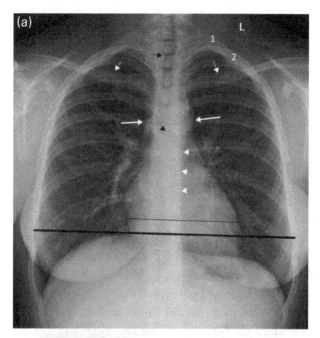

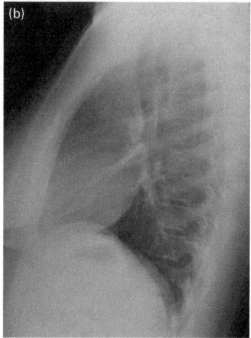

FIGURES 1.2a AND 1.2b. PA and lateral views of the chest in a normal 16-year-old for comparison (different patient). Note the normal appearance of structures. Contour of descending aorta (white arrowheads), superior mediastinal width between superior vena cava on the right and aortic arch on the left (white thick arrows on right and left side), tracheal air column (black arrow), carina (black arrowhead), and the orientation of the clavicles (thin white arrows). In a properly positioned patient the spinous processes lie midway between the medial ends of the clavicles. The cardiothoracic ratio is measured as the ratio of the cardiac transverse diameter (black thin line) divided by the maximum chest transverse diameter (thick black line). The first and second ribs on the left side are numbered (1, 2).

In general, electrocardiographic findings may include sinus tachycardia, dysrhythmia, low voltage, widened QRS, or repolarization abnormalities, with atrial or ventricular dysrhythmias leading to sudden death. Pathologic Q waves may be seen, and were found in one study with parvovirus B19 myocarditis.

Other tests that may help facilitate a timely diagnosis include a bedside ultrasound (US) for anatomic and functional evaluation, as well as assessment for pericardial fluid. This patient had an echocardiogram that showed a pericardial effusion, which was subsequently drained. A repeat chest radiograph shows the heart following the procedure (see Figure 1.1d).

Other tests that may be considered include creatine kinase MB, troponin, and BNP. Troponin I and troponin T, although not a sensitive or specific marker of myocarditis, may be elevated in acute myocarditis. Higher troponin levels have been associated with the need for extracorporeal membrane oxygenation (ECMO) and mortality. BNP and NT-proBNP are generally related to HF, not myocarditis, and are typically elevated and are associated with cardiac dysfunction and acute HF.

The chief complaints of adolescents with dilated cardiomyopathy following myocarditis rarely involve the cardiovascular system. The clinical presentation is characterized by multiple encounters with the healthcare system for nonspecific symptoms, antecedent viral infection, nonspecific respiratory and gastrointestinal symptoms, and fatigue which may or may not be exertional. The key symptom which is often overlooked or discounted is vague abdominal pain accompanied by nausea with minimal vomiting.

Dilated cardiomyopathy is notoriously difficult to diagnose in pediatrics. Young children often have chief complaints referable to the respiratory system, and adolescents present with abdominal pain. Therefore, a high index of suspicion is necessary to make an accurate diagnosis.

CASE CONCLUSIONS

In the current case, the patient's final diagnosis was dilated cardiomyopathy and pericardial effusion following myocarditis. He was admitted to the hospital, and an LVAD (left ventricular assist device) was placed 3 days later. He underwent cardiac transplant about 2 months later but unfortunately died due to accelerated rejection and infection shortly thereafter.

- Adolescents with cardiomyopathy/HF often have persistent, vague abdominal pain with minimal nausea and multiple visits.
- Young children with dilated cardiomyopathy often have respiratory symptoms such as tachypnea or wheezing.
- Patients with cardiomyopathy/HF may only have subtle signs of their disease and may rapidly decompensate.
- Cardiomyopathy and HF may predispose patients to fatal arrhythmias.
- Cardiac involvement in viral illnesses is common and may often go unnoticed. It can, in rare cases, have substantial acute hemodynamic and clinical sequelae, including pericardial effusion, dilated cardiomyopathy, and HF.

- Plain radiographs may be the first clue to the presence of a pericardial effusion, cardiomyopathy, or HF.
- Careful attention to the heart, mediastinum, airway, lungs, pleura, bones, and soft tissues on a pediatric chest x-ray is essential to accurately diagnose the cause of chest pain.
- Bedside US or an echocardiogram of the heart may reveal complications of myocarditis, including dilated cardiomyopathy and pericardial effusion.

Further Reading

1. Law YM, et al. Diagnosis and management of myocarditis in children: a scientific statement from the American Heart Association. *Circulation*. 2021;144:e123–e135. https://www.ahajournals.org/doi/10.1161/CIR.0000000000001001.

2 Fast-Breathing Baby

Ajay K. Puri, Mantosh S. Rattan, and Melissa A. McGuire

Case Study

A 7-day-old female patient is brought to your emergency department by ambulance for difficulty breathing. She was born via spontaneous vaginal delivery at 37 weeks gestation and had an uncomplicated hospital stay and was discharged at the end of day 2 post-delivery. Over the past day she began developing a cough and fever to 101°F, decreased feeding, and "fast breathing". Her vital signs are significant for a heart rate of 180 beats per minute, a rectal temperature of 102.1°F, a blood pressure of 78/44mmHg, a respiratory rate of 70 breaths per minute, and an oxygen saturation of 85% on room air. On physical examination she appears lethargic. She is tachypneic with retractions bilaterally, slightly dry mucous membranes, and coarse breath sounds over the right lower lobe. Despite supplemental oxygen via nasal cannula at 6 liters per minute, her oxygen saturation only increases to 91%. Her chest radiograph (CXR) is seen in Figure 2.1.

What do you do now?

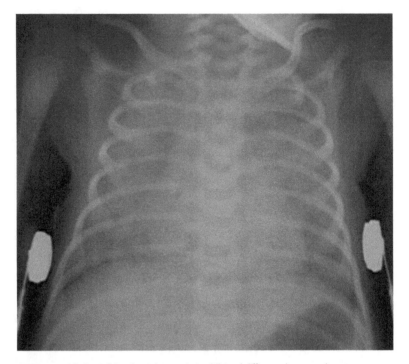

FIGURE 2.1. AP view of the chest demonstrates bilateral diffuse pulmonary air space opacification.

INTRODUCTION

Respiratory diseases are the leading conditions resulting in neonatal ICU admission in both preterm and term infants. Furthermore, respiratory distress of varying severity occurs in approximately 7% of neonates. As such, it is important for the emergency physician to be able to recognize and manage neonatal respiratory distress in its various presentations.

SIGNS AND SYMPTOMS

Signs of neonatal respiratory distress include:

- Tachypnea (respiratory rate >60 breaths per minute)
- Tachycardia (heart rate >160 beats per minute)

- Nasal flaring
- Grunting
- Chest wall retractions
- Cyanosis
- Apnea

Tachypnea is the most common presenting sign of a neonate in respiratory distress. Subtler symptoms include lethargy and poor feeding. Associated presenting signs may include hypothermia and hypoglycemia.

EMERGENCY MANAGEMENT

All neonates with respiratory distress should be placed on a continuous cardiac monitor and continuous pulse oximetry. Emergency management is directed at reversing hypoxia with oxygen supplementation and preventing or reversing respiratory acidosis by ensuring adequate ventilation. This may require support with humidified high flow nasal cannula (HHFNC) or with noninvasive positive pressure ventilation (NIPPV) such as continuous positive airway pressure (CPAP). Infants with evidence of upper airway obstruction with secretions should be suctioned beginning with a bulb-suction syringe. Patients with moderate to severe symptoms should have intravenous access obtained as they should be kept nil per os (NPO). Strong consideration to giving an initial bolus to replace losses already incurred should be made prior to starting maintenance intravenous fluids containing dextrose. A complete blood count, basic metabolic panel, a blood gas sample, and a CXR should also be performed to better determine the underlying pathology. There is a low threshold to begin antibiotic therapy in the ill-appearing infant with respiratory distress due to the difficulty in excluding bacterial infections.

Infants that are apneic, lose their airway protective reflexes such as a gag or cough, have continued respiratory failure despite NIPPV, or in whom chest compressions are started should be endotracheally intubated. Intubated patients will require contact with a tertiary care neonatal or pediatric intensive care team to assist with ventilator settings and/or for transfer to be arranged.

Neonatologists or pediatric intensivists should be involved early in the care of an ill neonate. A nonexhaustive list for when to involve a neonatologist for respiratory distress includes (adapted from Box 1 in Pramanik et al.):

- Inability to stabilize or ventilate an infant
- Requirement for vasopressors
- Cardiac disease suspected
- Meconium aspiration
- Sepsis with pneumonia
- Pneumothorax or pneumomediastinum.

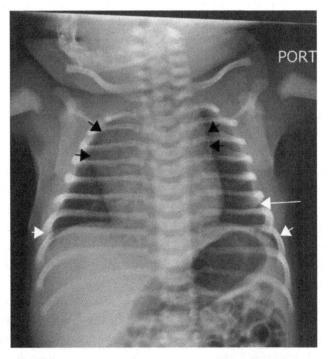

FIGURE 2.2. A normal neonatal chest radiograph. Note the sharp costophrenic angles (small white arrows), the aerated lung extending below the level of the 6th rib anteriorly (long white arrow), and the contour of a normal for age thymus expanding the superior mediastinum (small black arrows).

THE NORMAL NEONATAL CHEST RADIOGRAPH

The following should be evaluated systematically when approaching any neonatal CXR:

- Symmetric aeration—determined by visualization of the 6th rib anteriorly and 8th rib posteriorly
- Pulmonary vasculature—should be visible in the central 2/3 of the lungs
- Hemidiaphragm(s)—dome shaped with sharp costophrenic angles
- Cardiothoracic ratio can be up to 60% (0.6) in neonates. Cardiothoracic ratio is the ratio of maximal horizontal cardiac diameter to maximal horizontal thoracic diameter on a frontal CXR.
- Thymus gland
- Don't forget to evaluate the upper abdomen, bones, and soft tissues!

COMMON CONDITIONS PRESENTING AS NEONATAL RESPIRATORY DISTRESS

Transient Tachypnea of the Newborn

Transient tachypnea of the newborn (TTN) is the most common etiology of respiratory distress in neonates. It occurs in up to 6 per 1000 term births and 10 per 1000 preterm births. TTN may begin as early as 2 hours after delivery and last up to 5 days. Risk factors include maternal asthma, maternal diabetes, maternal sedation, fetal distress, delivery prior to 39 weeks gestation, and cesarean delivery.

Pathophysiology of TTN originates from delayed clearance and resorption of alveolar fluid from the intrauterine environment. During the stress of labor, release of fetal prostaglandins and adrenaline aid in the absorption of lung fluid. Cesarean delivery is thought to bypass this mechanism, thus increasing the risk for developing TTN.

CXR reflects the underlying pathophysiology, retained fetal lung fluid. This is seen in Figure 2.3 with interstitial opacities (thickening of the fissures and streaky opacities radiating from the hila), normal to increased lung volumes, and possibly small volume pleural fluid. A "prominent" cardiothymic silhouette may also be present. Blood gas measurements may

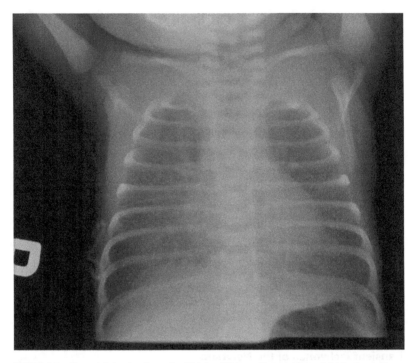

FIGURE 2.3. Neonatal chest radiograph with interstitial opacities and fissural thickening with normal to increase lung volumes suggestive of TTN.

show hypoxemia with normocarbia or hypercarbia with a mild respiratory acidosis.

However, definitive diagnosis often can only be made in retrospect once symptoms improve after a period of minimal intervention. Until then, overarching workup should include all possibilities.

Treatment of TTN is supportive. TTN usually responds to oxygen supplementation but may require CPAP to distend alveoli and support resorption of excess lung fluid. Mechanical ventilation is rarely required.

Pneumonia

Neonatal pneumonia can be divided into two categories; early onset (≤ 7 days) and late onset (> 7 days). Early onset (or congenital) pneumonia originates from transplacental infection or aspiration of infected amniotic fluid and usually presents within the first 72 hours of life. Group B streptococcus is the most common causative organism. Late onset pneumonia usually occurs after discharge; or, in the hospital, it is commonly acquired from the neonatal unit or is associated with mechanical ventilation.

Signs of neonatal pneumonia may mimic those of TTN and respiratory distress syndrome (RDS). Nonrespiratory signs include temperature instability, apnea, poor feeding, and lethargy. CXR can have protean imaging manifestations with radiographic findings potentially mimicking those seen in RDS, transient tachypnea of the newborn, and meconium aspiration. Isolated focal consolidation is rare with bilateral airspace disease most common, as seen in Figure 2.1. The presence of a pleural effusion can be a helpful distinguishing feature, being described in up to two-thirds of cases, such as in Figure 2.4.

Infants with suspected pneumonia require a full set of labs, including a complete blood count with a differential and blood cultures prior to initiating antibiotic therapy. It is worth noting that nearly all infants < 29 days

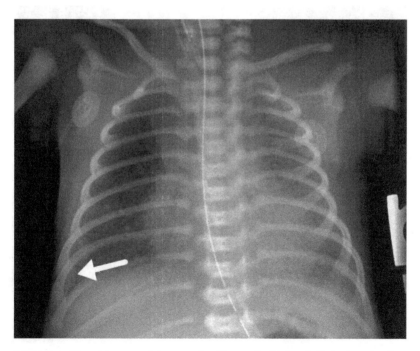

FIGURE 2.4. Neonatal pneumonia in a neonate with a small right pleural effusion (arrow) and diffuse left and right lower lobe hazy pulmonary opacification.

with a fever or hypothermia require a full septic workup, including a lumbar puncture.

Respiratory Distress Syndrome

RDS usually presents soon after birth and worsens over the following few hours. It is commonly observed in premature infants (< 37 weeks gestation) due to surfactant deficiency, with the risk of RDS decreasing as gestational age increases.

CXR reflects the underlying alveolar instability due to abnormal surface tension, demonstrating ground-glass/granular opacities and air bronchograms, as seen in Figure 2.5. Low lung volumes were classically described, but most neonates undergo imaging while under positive pressure support, often resulting in hyperinflation on the radiograph. Pleural effusions are not typical and may be an important clue to the possibility

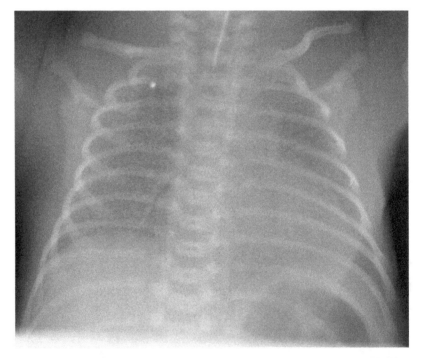

FIGURE 2.5. AP chest radiograph in a premature neonate with diffuse granular opacities. Endotracheal tube is present. Findings typical of respiratory distress syndrome (RDS).

of neonatal pneumonia. Air leak phenomena are common complications. Blood gas measurements demonstrate respiratory acidosis, hypoxemia, and eventually metabolic acidosis.

The cornerstone of management of RDS is prevention with antenatal corticosteroids. Routine administration of antenatal corticosteroids to mothers with threatened preterm birth has revolutionized the management of RDS. Neonates with mild to moderate presentations may respond to the distending forces of CPAP; however, severe cases require endotracheal intubation. Exogenous surfactant is routinely administered to preterm infants requiring endotracheal intubation at birth to prevent RDS.

Pneumothorax

Spontaneous pneumothorax occurs in about 1%–2% of term infants. Risk factors include premature births, meconium aspiration, and RDS. This is likely due to their requirement for positive pressure ventilation which can lead to an air leak, causing the creation of a pneumothorax.

On physical examination, decreased breath sounds may be auscultated on the side of the pneumothorax. CXR demonstrates a lack of lung markings and lucency in the hemithorax with the pneumothorax. Decubitus films can better depict the findings as opposed to supine films, as seen in Figure 2.6. The neonate is lying in the left lateral decubitus position to reflect a right-sided pneumothorax.

Signs of a tension pneumothorax may include contralateral tracheal deviation, jugular venous distention, hypoxia, cyanosis, and/or hemodynamic instability. Tension pneumothoraces should be decompressed emergently.

Management of pneumothoraces depends on severity. If the patient is alert, has an oxygen saturation above 90%, and has normal vital signs, consult a pediatric surgeon or neonatologist to discuss placement of a pigtail catheter or chest tube. These may resolve spontaneously without intervention if the positive pressure that likely led to its creation is withdrawn. However, a chest tube should be placed immediately if the patient decompensates.

Meconium Aspiration Syndrome

Meconium aspiration syndrome (MAS) is usually a sequela of fetal distress during labor. Fetal distress may lead to passage of meconium. Fetal distress

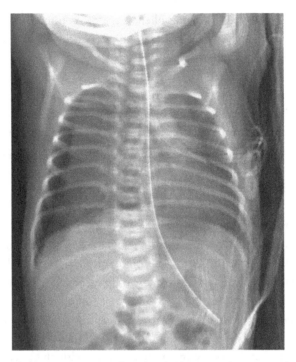

FIGURE 2.6. Left lateral decubitus view of the chest in this neonate demonstrates the peripheral lucency and lack of lung markings in the right chest, consistent with right-sided pneumothorax.

may also cause a gasping respiratory effort, leading to aspiration of meconium. Not all infants born with stained amniotic fluid will have MAS. An estimated 13% of live births involve meconium-stained amniotic fluid, and only 4%–5% of these will develop MAS. MAS requiring mechanical ventilation has a reported 6.6% mortality.

MAS is suspected in the infant born with meconium-stained amniotic fluid accompanied by respiratory distress in the few hours after birth. Meconium is extremely toxic to the lungs of a newborn due to acidity, causing airway inflammation, deactivation of surfactant, chemical pneumonitis, and mechanical obstruction. CXR reflects the underlying bronchial obstruction and chemical pneumonitis. This may range from generalized hyperinflation to the classic patchy, coarse, and asymmetric disease due to intermixed areas of focal hyperinflation and

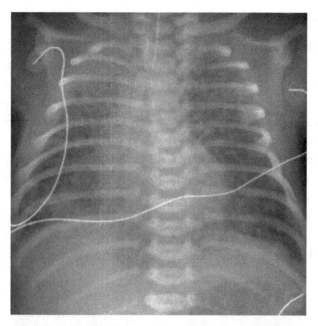

FIGURE 2.7. CXR in a neonate born with meconium-stained amniotic fluid demonstrates patchy coarse bilateral air space pulmonary opacification, in addition to generalized hyperinflation.

atelectasis, as seen in Figure 2.7. Air-leak phenomena are commonly encountered.

In the past, oropharyngeal and nasopharyngeal suctioning was performed on the meconium-stained infant after delivery of the head (but before the shoulders) as it was thought to prevent aspiration. It is no longer recommended, as it does not reduce the incidence of MAS. Vigorous infants should receive bulb syringe suctioning and respiratory support with supplemental oxygen and CPAP as required. Routine endotracheal suctioning of infants is no longer recommended.

When MAS is suspected, broad-spectrum antibiotic therapy is necessary, as meconium is a medium for growth of gram-negative organisms. Infants with severe MAS will require transfer to a tertiary center capable of administering surfactant, high-frequency ventilation, inhaled nitric oxide, and/or initiating extracorporeal membrane oxygenation (ECMO).

UNCOMMON DIAGNOSES

Congenital Diaphragmatic Hernia

Congenital diaphragmatic hernias (CDHs) affect one in 2500 live births. It is due to a failure of a portion of the diaphragm to develop during embryological formation, leading to herniation of abdominal contents into the thorax. This adversely affects lung growth and alveolar development. Antenatal diagnosis is made in only 59% of cases.

Diagnosis is usually made on CXR performed for the neonate in respiratory distress; 85% of CDHs occur on the left. The radiographic appearance depends on the contents and amount of gas within the herniated bowel. Lung hypoplasia is present, including the unaffected side. Figure 2.8 depicts a left-sided CDH, while Figure 2.9 depicts a right sided CDH.

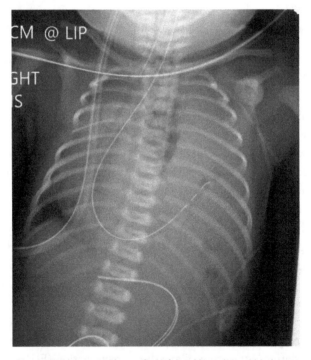

FIGURE 2.8. Neonatal chest x-ray with opacified left hemithorax into which the stomach has herniated, resulting in malpositioned enteric tube and midline shift to the right, in this patient with a left-sided CDH.

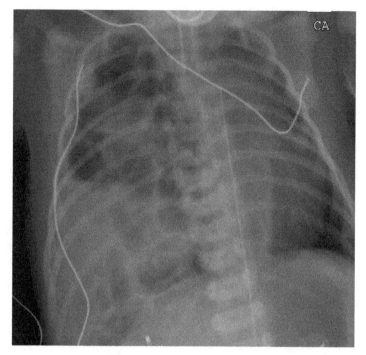

FIGURE 2.9. Neonate with multiple bubbly lucencies corresponding to bowel loops and a higher density corresponding to liver occupying the right hemithorax in this patient with a right-sided CDH.

The defect requires surgical correction after the patient has been stabilized medically. A pediatric surgeon should be consulted. If a CDH is diagnosed antenatally, the patient should be transferred to be managed in a perinatal center.

Tracheoesophageal Fistula/Esophageal Atresia

Tracheoesophageal fistula (TEF) and esophageal atresia (EA) occur in about 1 in 2500 births. It is a spectrum of disease due to incomplete/abnormal division of the foregut. The majority of cases are the proximal esophageal atresia with a distal fistula subtype, while isolated esophageal atresia is the next most common. Antenatally there may have been polyhydramnios and a small stomach on ultrasound. Clinically, the infant presents with drooling and choking with attempted feeding. In all subtypes of EA/TEF except the

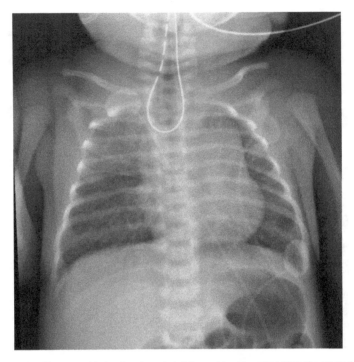

FIGURE 2.10. Neonate with drooling. An enteric tube could not be passed into the stomach and the tube coiled in the proximal esophagus in this patient with TEF and EA. Distal air in the stomach implies a distal TE fistula.

H-type, the attempted passage of an enteric tube will not be successful with the tube coiled in the proximal esophagus (seen in Figure 2.10). The presence of air in the stomach and bowel in this setting implies a distal fistula.

Diagnosis is usually made after birth. Respiratory issues are usually related to aspiration of secretions either from the esophageal pouch or via the TEF. The H-type fistula usually presents later in the infancy with recurring episodes of aspiration. Surgical correction of the fistula is definitive management.

Other Considerations

It is important to remember that not all neonatal respiratory distress is pulmonary in origin. Congenital heart defects (CHD) occur in about 1% of births annually and may present with respiratory distress. Cyanotic heart disease in a newborn may present with an intense cyanosis that is disproportionate to their respiratory distress and a lack of improvement in oxygen saturation when 100% oxygen has been supplied. CHD may also be suggested by an infant with an audible murmur on cardiac exam, or decreased femoral pulses and lower extremity pulses as in aortic coarctation. Chest X-ray and electrocardiography might allude to congenital structural abnormalities which can usually be confirmed on echocardiography.

Case Conclusion

The patient was diagnosed with diffuse bilateral pneumonia, leading to sepsis and hypoxic respiratory failure. She was bulb suctioned, given rectal acetaminophen, and placed on nasal CPAP at a pressure of $5cmH_2O$ and FiO2 40%, with improvement in her oxygenation to 95%. Her tachypnea improved to 55 breaths per minute and her tachycardia improved to 162 beats per minute. Intravenous access was obtained, blood cultures were drawn, and she was given ampicillin and gentamicin for antimicrobial coverage. She was given a bolus of normal saline, followed by maintenance fluids with dextrose 5% normal saline. A lumbar puncture did not reveal evidence of meningitis. She was admitted to the pediatric intensive care unit for further management.

KEY POINTS

- Recognizing neonatal respiratory distress is the first important step; tachypnea (RR > 60 breaths per minute), tachycardia (bpm > 160 beats per minute), grunting, stridor, chest wall retractions, cyanosis, and apnea are all indications of respiratory distress that should be addressed.
- Involve a neonatologist or pediatric intensivist early in your resuscitation of a neonate in respiratory distress, particularly those requiring NIPPV or endotracheal intubation.
- Not all respiratory distress is pulmonary in origin. Consider sepsis or congenital heart disease in the patients differential.
- Regardless of the cause of the respiratory distress, a febrile infant below 28 days old should undergo a full septic workup,

including lumbar puncture, blood cultures, and empiric broad spectrum antibiotics.
· In a neonate with significant respiratory distress requiring support, consider empiric antibiotics, as presentations of many benign pathologies such as TTN can overlap with bacterial pneumonia.

TIPS FROM THE RADIOLOGIST

· Always use a systematic approach for evaluation of the CXR.
· Make sure there is symmetric aeration: 6th rib anterior/8th rib posterior.
· Check the pulmonary vasculature—visible in the central 2/3 of the lungs.
· Assess the hemidiaphragm(s)—dome shaped/sharp costophrenic angles.
· Assess the transverse cardiothoracic ratio—up to 60% in neonates.
· Evaluate the thymus.
· Don't forget to evaluate the upper abdomen, bones, and soft tissues!

Further Reading

1. Gershel J, Crain E, Cunningham S, Meltzer J. *Clinical Manual of Emergency Pediatrics*. 6th ed. Cambridge: Cambridge University Press; 2018:1–36, 760–761.
2. Suprenant S, Coghlan M. Respiratory distress in the newborn: An approach for the emergency care provider. *Clin Pediatr Emerg Med*. 2016;17(2):113–121. https://doi.org/10.1016/j.cpem.2016.03.004.
3. Gallacher D, Hart K, Kotecha S. Common respiratory conditions of the newborn. *Breathe*. 2016;12(1):30–42. https://doi.org/10.1183/20734735.000716.
4. Hermansen CL, Mahajan A. Newborn respiratory distress. *Am Fam Physician*. 2015 Dec 1;92(11):994–1002. PMID: 26760414.
5. Reuter S, Moser C, Baack M. Respiratory distress in the newborn. *Pediatr Rev*. 2014 Oct;35(10):417–28; quiz 429. doi: 10.1542/pir.35-10-417. PMID: 25274969; PMCID: PMC4533247.
6. Pramanik AK, Rangaswamy N, Gates T. Neonatal respiratory distress: A practical approach to its diagnosis and management. *Pediatr Clin North Am*. 2015 Apr;62(2):453–69. doi: 10.1016/j.pcl.2014.11.008. PMID: 25836708.

3 Green Vomit . . . Ewwww!!!

Esther Ro, Yamini Jadcherla, and Maegan S. Reynolds

Case Study

A mother brings her 18-day-old male infant to the emergency department for vomiting. The baby was born at 36 weeks after an uncomplicated pregnancy via spontaneous vaginal delivery. At birth, the APGARS were 8 and 9, with no neonatal resuscitation required. The baby weighed 6 pounds 7 ounces and was discharged by 48 hours. Meconium passed within the first 24 hours of life. The infant has been tolerating breast milk but having small spit-ups; his mother was told that these were due to reflux. However, over the past 12 hours, he has had increased vomiting, which is now a dark brown/green color. The baby is fussier and not as interested in feeding. He is voiding and stooling at baseline. He has no fevers or respiratory symptoms. He is afebrile, heart rate is 175 beats per minute and regular, respiratory rate is 45 breaths per minute, and he has an oxygen saturation of 98% on room air. Physical exam is notable for a fussy infant with a distended abdomen and decreased bowel sounds. He has capillary refill of 3–4 seconds and increased skin turgor.

What do you do now?

DIAGNOSIS/DISCUSSION

The clinician should begin immediate volume resuscitation and obtain radiographic imaging. In an ill-appearing infant with delayed capillary refill and increased skin turgor, an IV should be placed, and labs including a complete blood count, chemistries, and blood cultures should be obtained. An IV fluid bolus of normal saline (NS) or lactate ringers (LR) at 20 ml/kg should be given, and additional boluses may be needed based on the infant's exam and vital signs.

An abdominal radiograph (AXR) was obtained (Figure 3.1), which is negative for free air, but has other concerning findings.

Additional interventions include gastric decompression with a nasogastric tube and pediatric surgery consultation. Given the bilious emesis, the clinician was appropriately concerned for malrotation with

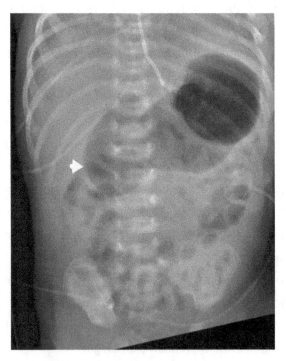

FIGURE 3.1. Abdominal radiograph demonstrates dilatation of the stomach and proximal duodenum (arrowhead). Distal gas is present in nondilated bowel loops.

midgut volvulus (MGV), and an upper gastrointestinal (UGI) fluoroscopy series was obtained (Figure 3.2a), which confirms the diagnosis of malrotation with MGV. Contrast this with Figure 3.2b which demonstrates a normal UGI.

Emergent surgical evaluation was obtained, and the patient was taken to the OR for a Ladd's procedure. If a neonatal UGI or pediatric surgery consultation is not immediately available at the facility, the neonate should be transferred to a tertiary pediatric hospital where advanced imaging and pediatric surgery are available. Surgery via the Ladd's procedure is necessary to reduce the volvulus and reduce the risk for recurrent volvulus. However, long-term complications, including small bowel obstruction, short gut syndrome, or recurrent volvulus, may occur in patients with a congenital malrotation.

The key for the clinical provider is correctly eliciting a history of bilious emesis. Bilious emesis in a neonate is always pathologic and a sign of intestinal obstruction (mechanical or functional) until proven otherwise. The differential diagnosis for bilious emesis in a neonate should include duodenal atresia, intestinal malrotation, volvulus causing obstruction, jejunoileal atresia, necrotizing enterocolitis, meconium ileus, or Hirschsprung's disease. Alternatively, nonbilious emesis in a neonate is often benign, related to overfeeding or reflux, or may be due to hypertrophic pyloric stenosis or an infectious etiology such as acute viral gastroenteritis. However, any bilious emesis is concerning and further emergent workup is warranted.

Malrotation occurs secondary to failure of normal gut development in the 4th to 8th week of gestation. Always assess for comorbid conditions or anomalies with a diagnosis of malrotation, which are present in more than 50% of cases. The most frequent include congenital diaphragmatic hernia, congenital heart disease, and Trisomy 21. Young infants usually present with bilious emesis, but may also present with progression and complications including peritonitis from perforation, shock, or hematochezia from bowel wall necrosis related to the volvulus. Diagnosis after 1 year of age is often due to evaluation for failure to thrive, malabsorption, cyclic vomiting syndrome, or chronic diarrhea. Additionally, bilious emesis in the older child can be related to progressive acute gastroenteritis, intussusception, peritonitis, or appendicitis.

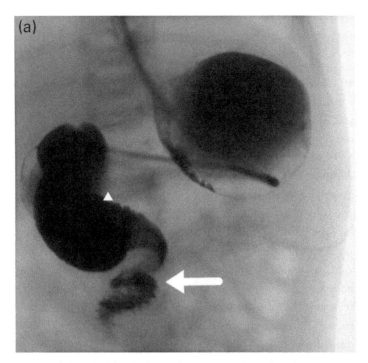

FIGURE 3.2a. UGI shows the dilated proximal duodenum (arrowhead) and the corkscrew configuration of the duodenum (arrow), which is diagnostic for MGV.

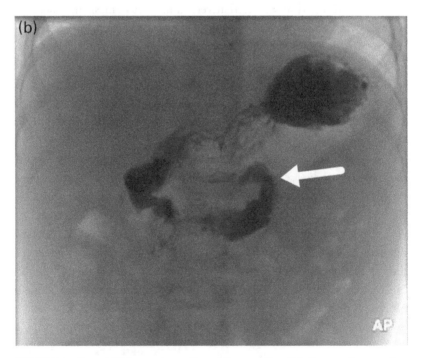

FIGURE 3.2b. Normal UGI in a newborn with nonbilious vomiting. Note the normal course of duodenum with the duodenojejunal junction (arrow) to the left of midline reaching the level of the first part of duodenum and pylorus.

An AXR is a bedside imaging modality that may be used to rule out perforation, particularly as it can be done at the bedside in an unstable patient.

The AXR can demonstrate radiographic signs of proximal obstruction in a child with MGV. The stomach can be disproportionately distended compared to distal bowel (Figure 3.3).

Although MGV occurs distal to the gastric outlet, the duodenum is slower to distend in the acute setting. There is usually a paucity of distal bowel gas, but this can vary depending on the severity and duration of the obstruction. With prolonged obstruction, more likely from Ladd bands, the duodenum can distend to create a double bubble pattern with distal gas (Figure 3.1).

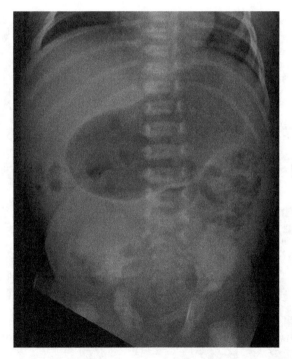

FIGURE 3.3. Abdominal radiograph of 7-day-old male with bilious emesis and midgut volvulus. The stomach is disproportionately distended compared to the distal bowel gas. The duodenum is not visualized. This pattern can be benign at any age; but one should consider MGV in the setting of bilious emesis.

The presence of distal gas distinguishes this pattern from the true double bubble without distal gas, which is diagnostic for duodenal atresia (Figure 3.4).

The presence of a decompressing nasogastric tube or frequent vomiting may alter the bowel gas pattern and make it appear normal. Other causes of proximal bowel obstruction can present with similar bowel gas patterns; for example, duodenal stenosis or web and annular pancreas.

The first-line imaging exam to diagnose malrotation and MGV is the fluoroscopic UGI series. The AXR in a child with MGV can be deceivingly normal without evidence for obstruction. A normal AXR should not reassure the clinician in an infant with bilious emesis, and further workup with a UGI should be performed.

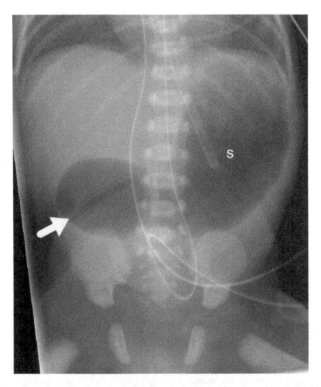

FIGURE 3.4. Zero-day-old male in the NICU. Classic double bubble sign without distal bowel gas, diagnostic for duodenal atresia. Dilated duodenum (arrow). Dilated stomach (S).

Additional radiographic patterns on AXR require special mention. Diffuse bowel dilatation or multiple dilated and separated loops of bowel are ominous findings in a sick child with bilious emesis and peritoneal signs (Figure 3.5 and Figures 3.6a and 3.6b). These patterns should raise concern for bowel ischemia or infarction secondary to MGV and vascular compromise.

An UGI should be performed to differentiate MGV from these other etiologies and prompt urgent intervention. The UGI requires administration of an oral contrast agent to delineate the anatomy of the duodenum under fluoroscopy. The average effective dose of ionizing radiation in the UGI in a neonate is 1.6 to 3.2 mSv. This dose is approximate to 1 year of

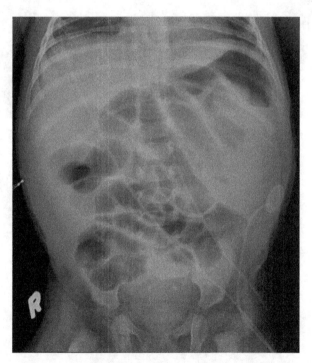

FIGURE 3.5. Abdominal radiograph of 7-week-old female with bilious emesis and midgut volvulus. There is dilatation of multiple loops of bowel throughout the abdomen. In the appropriate clinical setting, ileus can be a sign of bowel ischemia resulting from MGV. Functional obstruction of prematurity or a distal bowel obstruction can present with a similar bowel gas pattern in neonates.

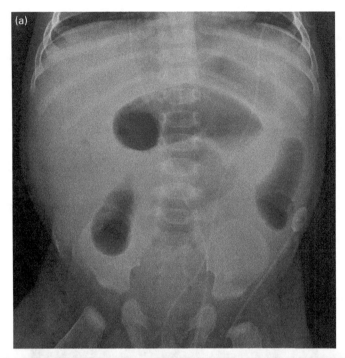

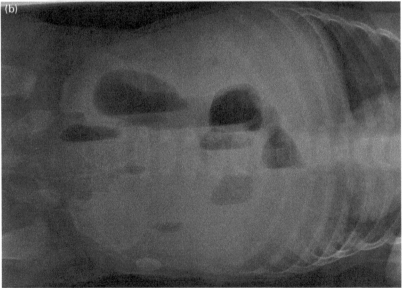

FIGURES 3.6a AND 3.6b. Four-month-old male with bilious emesis and midgut volvulus. AP supine (a) and left lateral decubitus (b) abdominal radiographs. Dilated small bowel loops with air fluid levels are separated and scattered in the abdomen. In a very ill child with bilious emesis, this bowel gas pattern should raise concern for an ominous intra-abdominal pathology, such as MGV with bowel ischemia or infarction.

natural background radiation in the United States, which is 3 mSv. The normal duodenum on the UGI is posterior in course, which infers a retroperitoneal position, and the duodenojejunal junction is located to the left of the vertebral pedicles and as high as the duodenal bulb. Malrotation is diagnosed when these criteria are not met. MGV is diagnosed when there is a corkscrew course of the duodenum, which mirrors the twisting of the bowel around the vascular pedicle (Figure 3.2a). When there is a tight volvulus, there is complete obstruction of contrast with a beaklike appearance of the duodenum at the point of obstruction.

Malrotation and MGV can be diagnosed on ultrasonography and computed tomography (CT); in fact, there are a few select institutions where US is the first-line exam for MGV. Ultrasound (US) may be the first exam performed if there is initial concern for hypertrophic pyloric stenosis. On US, an inverted relationship between the superior mesenteric artery and vein, where the vein is to the left of the artery, is suspicious for malrotation, and the duodenum should be carefully evaluated by US or should prompt an UGI. On US, an intraperitoneal course of the transverse duodenum is diagnostic for malrotation. The whirlpool sign, which represents the twisting of bowel and mesentery around the vascular pedicle, is diagnostic for volvulus. Similar findings can be seen on abdominal CT.

Ultimately, once the clinician has astutely recognized the concerning feature of bilious emesis in a neonate, further workup must be obtained. The clinician should continue with bedside resuscitation including IV fluids, gastric decompression, and close monitoring with serial abdominal exams. While an AXR may show some signs of obstruction or volvulus, other than to rule out perforation with free air, an AXR is not diagnostic. All neonates with bilious emesis should have an UGI performed. If an UGI is not available, the clinician should transfer the infant to a tertiary care center for further workup. Once the diagnosis of malrotation is made, treatment is through a Ladd's procedure by a pediatric surgeon.

- The triad of bilious emesis, abdominal pain, and distension is pathologic and indicates intestinal obstruction, either mechanical or functional, thus warranting further workup. Neonates may not always present with all these findings.
- Initial resuscitation includes gastric decompression via NG tube and IV fluids.

- The AXR findings for MGV are nonspecific and can vary from normal to diffuse bowel dilatation. A normal bowel gas pattern should not be reassuring.
- The fluoroscopic UGI series is typically the first-line imaging exam to diagnose or rule out MGV. An abnormal duodenal course with a corkscrew pattern or a beak-like obstruction of the second portion of duodenum are seen with MGV on UGI study.
- Pathognomonic radiographic signs on a plain radiograph include double bubble sign for duodenal atresia (no distal bowel gas).
- Reversed SMA/SMV relationship on US is suspicious for malrotation and should prompt workup. A whirlpool sign on US is diagnostic for volvulus.

Further Reading

1. Applegate KE. Evidence-based diagnosis of malrotation and volvulus. *Pediatr Radiol.* 2009;39(Suppl 2):S161–S163. https://doi.org/10.1007/s00247-009-1177-x.
2. Brandt ML. Intestinal malrotation in children. In: Post TW, ed. *UpToDate.* UpToDate, Waltham, MA: UpToDate. Accessed April 30, 2021.
3. Burge DM. The management of bilious vomiting in the neonate. *Early Hum Dev.* 2016;102:41–45. doi:10.1016/j.earlhumdev.2016.09.002.
4. Damilakis J, Stratakis J, Raissaki M, Perisinakis K, Kourbetis N, Gourtsoyiannis N. (2006). Normalized dose data for upper gastrointestinal tract contrast studies performed to infants. *Med Phys.* 2006;33(4):1033–1040. https://aapm.onlinelibr ary.wiley.com/doi/abs/10.1118/1.2181297.
5. Kimura K, Loening-Baucke V. Bilious vomiting in the newborn: rapid diagnosis of intestinal obstruction. *Am Fam Physician.* 2000;61(9):2791–2798.

6. Maxfield CM, Bartz BH, Shaffer JL. A pattern-based approach to bowel obstruction in the newborn. *Pediatr Radiol.* 2013;43(3):318–329. https://doi.org/10.1007/s00247-012-2573-1.
7. Nehra D, Goldstein AM. Intestinal malrotation: varied clinical presentation from infancy through adulthood. *Surgery.* 2011;149:386.
8. Ooms N, Matthyssens LE, Draaisma JM, et al. Laparoscopic treatment of intestinal malrotation in children. *Eur J Pediatr Surg.* 2016;26:376.
9. Staton, RJ, Williams JL, Arreola MM, Hintenlang DE, Bolch WE. (2007). Organ and effective doses in infants undergoing upper gastrointestinal (UGI) fluoroscopic examination. *Med Phys.* 2007;34(2):703–710. https://aapm.onlinelibrary.wiley.com/doi/abs/10.1118/1.2426405.

4 What's That in the Diaper?

Maegan S. Reynolds, Yamini Jadcherla, and Esben Vogelius

Case Study

A mother brings in her 12-day-old female infant to the Emergency Department (ED) for bloody stools. She was born at 37 weeks via assisted vaginal delivery due to maternal gestational hypertension. The infant had APGARs of 9 and 9, required no resuscitation, and was discharged within 48 hours of delivery. She has been tolerating breastfeeding and has regular yellow seedy stools. For the past few days she has been fussier and not wanting to feed. On the day of presentation, her stools became dark and foul smelling, and her last two stools had frank blood. The infant has had no fevers, cyanosis or difficulty breathing, but has had minimal urine output today. On arrival she is afebrile, heart rate is 180 beats per minute, respiratory rate is 48 breaths per minute, with an oxygen saturation of 97% on room air. On physical examination the infant is fussy even when being held. Her extremities are mottled, with capillary refill of 3–4 seconds. She has a firm distended abdomen with decreased bowel sounds and diffuse tenderness.

What do you do now?

DISCUSSION

Parents of neonates are very focused on their infants' ins and outs, particularly with what they see in the diaper. It is not uncommon for parents of neonates to present to the ED, asking for your opinion on their infants' stools, frequently bringing the offending diaper in to show the provider. While rectal bleeding in infants can be from benign conditions, it can be a marker of serious illness, as with the ill-appearing neonate described in this case.

The differential diagnosis of bloody stools varies by age, even within the pediatric population. Many conditions can occur at any age, such as infectious colitis, vascular malformations, or anal fissures. Certain etiologies are more common in toddlers, such as Meckel's diverticulum, intussusception, or hemolytic uremic syndrome (HUS). Other etiologies, such as inflammatory bowel disease, are more common in school-age children. In neonates the worrisome diagnoses include necrotizing enterocolitis (NEC), malrotation with volvulus, coagulopathies, Hirschsprung's disease, and infectious colitis. Less concerning causes include swallowed maternal blood either from delivery or breastfeeding from a cracked nipple, anal fissures, or a milk-protein allergy. If the infant is toxic appearing with a distended tender abdomen and signs of shock, presume the infant has an emergent condition and initiate prompt resuscitation and workup.

While uncommon, bowel hypoperfusion due to congenital heart disease (CHD) can also lead to bloody stools. If the history and physical is suggestive of CHD, consider smaller fluid boluses such as 10ml/kg. If the patient requires large volume resuscitation perform frequent reassessments for signs of heart failure, such as a gallop or hepatomegaly. Labs such as a complete blood count (CBC), coagulation studies such as PT/PTT/INR, lactate, and chemistries should be obtained. Also, consider disseminated intravascular coagulopathy (DIC) labs and infectious stool studies (for pathogens such as shigella or salmonella). Also consider coagulopathies in those with a family history of bleeding disorders, or prolonged bleeding after umbilical stump detachment or circumcision. If the infant did not receive vitamin K after birth, they can present with bloody stools and should be treated with IV vitamin K on presentation.

NEC is caused by ischemic necrosis of the intestine, leading to inflammation and entrance of gas-forming organisms into the bowel wall. NEC is most common in premature low-birth-weight infants, and less than 10% occurs in full-term infants. NEC is most commonly diagnosed in the neonatal intensive care unit (NICU) with a change in feeding tolerance. It most commonly presents in the ED with bloody stools, abdominal distension, and feeding intolerance with emesis. In full-term infants it usually presents within the first 2 weeks of life, and one must consider a predisposing condition such as sepsis or congenital heart disease. NEC is associated with high morbidity, in the short term with shock, DIC, or sepsis, and long-term complications such as short gut syndrome, strictures, adhesion ileus, or bowel obstruction. Mortality is inversely proportional to gestational age, with ~40% mortality in early preterm infants and ~10% mortality in term infants. Surgical management increases mortality, and about 50% of infants will have long-term sequelae such as short gut syndrome.

Once the diagnosis of NEC is made, the ED provider should focus on resuscitation. Providers should ensure adequate IV access and administer IV fluids to improve signs of shock, correct dehydration, and support blood pressure. Given this neonate's signs of shock with mottling and delayed capillary refill, the provider should immediately obtain IV access and give IV fluid resuscitation with 20ml/kg crystalloid bolus. NEC also leads to bowel wall inflammation and capillary leak, so continued IV fluids are needed. The infant should have bowel rest with all enteral feeding stopped. Additionally, placement of a nasogastric tube for gastric emptying and decompression assists with bowel rest. Empiric broad spectrum antibiotics such as ampicillin, gentamicin, and metronidazole combination or piperacillin-tazobactam and gentamicin combination should be initiated immediately. If able, blood cultures should be obtained prior to starting antibiotics. Additional supportive care should continue, such as respiratory support with intubation and mechanical ventilation, cardiovascular support with vasopressors, correcting electrolyte or metabolic derangements, or treating thrombocytopenia, anemia, or DIC.

Additionally, all neonates with NEC should have a surgical consultation. While most can be managed medically with bowel rest, antibiotics, resuscitation, and parenteral nutrition, surgical intervention may be necessary in up to 50% of cases. Indications for surgical intervention vary. Pneumoperitoneum is the most commonly accepted indication for surgery. Surgical options include laparotomy in the operating room versus peritoneal drainage placement at the bedside. Infants should be admitted to a closely monitored setting, likely to an ICU initially. The need for pediatric or neonatal ICU admission or pediatric surgical consultation may necessitate the need for transfer to a tertiary care pediatric hospital.

The choice of imaging for bloody stools is related to the most likely diagnosis and age of the patient. In young infants, NEC or malrotation with volvulus must be excluded as the etiology for bloody stools, and the initial imaging of choice is an abdominal x-ray. In toxic appearing neonates, x-ray is easily obtained at the bedside, but should be considered in well-appearing neonates without another identifiable cause. In our case, an abdominal x-ray was obtained and showed pneumatosis and portal venous gas, confirming the suspected diagnosis of NEC.

Findings to look for on abdominal radiographs with concern for NEC include pneumatosis, bowel dilation, portal venous gas, or free air. A degree of bowel dilation is seen in a majority (~90%) of patients with NEC. While bowel dilation is a nonspecific finding, the degree of dilation tends to correlate with the severity of disease. Abdominal radiographs are also followed regularly in patients undergoing medical treatment for NEC to assess for change. A localized or fixed pattern of dilation on serial radiographs raises concern for bowel necrosis. Pneumatosis is a specific imaging finding that confirms the clinical diagnosis of NEC, though it is variably present ranging from 19%–98% of cases. The extent of pneumatosis does not always correlate with severity of disease and can resolve rapidly. Pneumatosis can be bubbly or linear in morphology on radiographs with submucosal or subserosal distribution of bowel wall air. Portal venous gas is typically a later sign seen in up to 30% of patients with NEC. It is typically seen in more clinically severe cases (Figures 4.1a and 4.1b). Free air is the most common indication for immediate surgical intervention. Free air typically results from a perforation in the distal ileum or colon. While pneumoperitoneum can be detected on supine radiographs, a cross-table lateral or left lateral decubitus radiograph increases the sensitivity for detecting small amounts of free air (Figure 4.2).

Ultrasound (US) is emerging as a complementary imaging modality in infants with NEC. While not as commonly used, US can visualize the same findings seen on x-ray. Additionally, US allows for the evaluation of bowel wall thickness, echogenicity, peristalsis, perfusion, and detection of free fluid or focal intra-abdominal fluid collections.

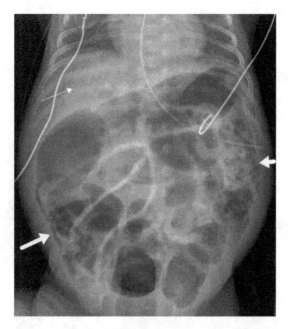

FIGURE 4.1a. Necrotizing enterocolitis (NEC) with pneumatosis and portal venous gas. Three-week-old male, ex-27-weeker, with tender distended abdomen and metabolic acidosis. Radiograph shows classic linear morphology of subserosal pneumatosis in the right abdomen (long white arrow) and bubbly morphology of submucosal pneumatosis in the left abdomen (short white arrow). Additionally, branching air is noted in the right upper quadrant, consistent with coexistent portal venous gas (thin white arrow).

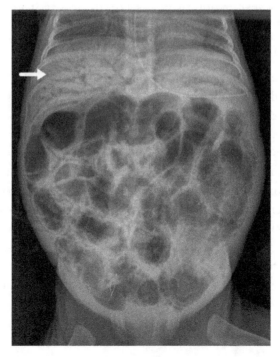

FIGURE 4.1b. After multiple surgical interventions and extensive bowel resection there was progression of diffuse pneumatosis and extensive portal venous gas (white arrow).

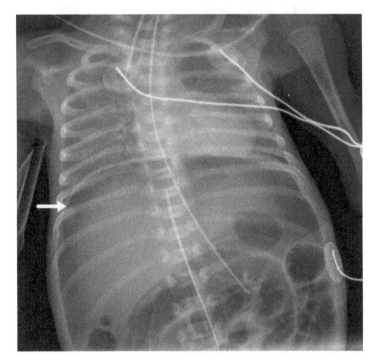

FIGURE 4.2.   Necrotizing enterocolitis (NEC) presenting with free air and progressive pneumatosis and portal venous gas. Three-day-old 28-week premature infant. Extensive upper abdominal free air was discovered on portable chest x-ray. This outlines the hemidiaphragms (white arrow) and distends the abdomen. No pneumatosis or portal venous gas was radiographically evident at this time.

Additional imaging to consider in older children presenting with bloody stools includes ultrasound for intussusception. The classic presentation for intussusception is an infant to toddler with intermittent episodes of severe abdominal pain who later develops bloody stools. Intussusception usually presents between ages 6 to 36 months of age, and less than 1% occur in infants under 3 months of age. Ultrasound is the screening modality of choice for ileocolic intussusception (Figures 4.3a and 4.3b). It has excellent diagnostic performance with both high sensitivity (98%–100%) and specificity (88%–100%) for the diagnosis. Radiographs alone have a much lower sensitivity (45%) and cannot reliably exclude the diagnosis of intussusception. However, there is added value in abdominal radiographs

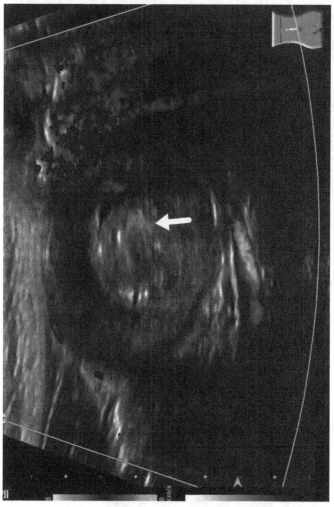

FIGURE 4.3a. Ileocolic intussusception. Four-month-old female with abdominal pain and vomiting. Ultrasound shows the typical targetoid appearance of the intussusception in the short axis (axial). The internal echogenicity represents internal herniated mesenteric fat (white arrow).

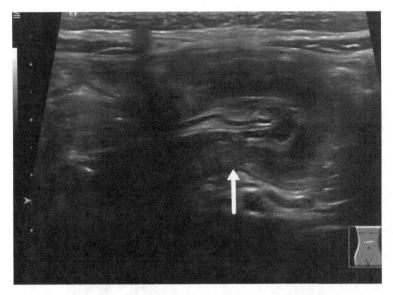

FIGURE 4.3b. Longitudinal image of the intussusception in long axis (sagittal). This appearance has been described as kidney-like in appearance.

to evaluate for obstruction and exclude pneumoperitoneum, which is a contraindication to enema reduction. Fluoroscopic enema has a high sensitivity and specificity for the diagnosis of intussusception (approaching 100%) (Figure 4.4). However, given the more invasive nature of the exam

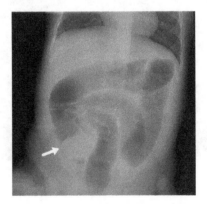

FIGURE 4.4. Fluoroscopic save image during air enema reduction of intussusception with intussusception now seen in the cecum (arrow). Initial intussusception was seen in the transverse colon during the study.

and the associated radiation, this is now almost exclusively reserved for treatment. As a therapeutic modality, enema demonstrates a high non-surgical reduction rate (74.1%–79.6%) and low complication rate (perforation rate of 0.6%–0.8%). Patients who fail enema reduction require surgical reduction, with 20%–40% of this subset of patients ultimately requiring bowel resection.

A Meckel's diverticulum must also be considered in children with bloody stools but is rarely diagnosed in the neonate. The classic teaching is that Meckel's occurs in 2% of the population, occurs within 2 feet of the ileocecal valve, is 2 inches in length, contains 2 types of tissues including ectopic tissues such as gastric mucosa, and presents before the age of 2. Meckel's can present in children with painless lower gastrointestinal bleeding or hematochezia. However, it can also incidentally be found due to complications including an intussusception lead point, perforation with pneumoperitoneum, bowel obstruction, or clinical history and exam

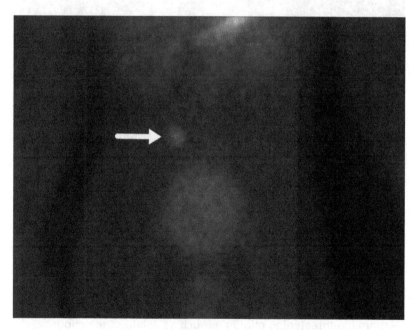

FIGURE 4.5a. Meckel's diverticulum. Five-year-old child with bloody stools and lower abdominal pain. Planar image from Technetium-99m pertechnetate scan (Meckel scan) shows focal abnormal uptake in the right lower quadrant (white arrow). Expected gastric update and bladder excretion are also seen.

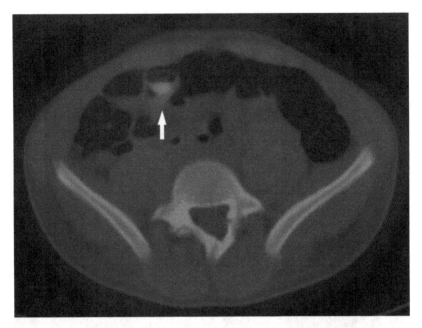

FIGURE 4.5b. Uptake can be better localized with CT fusion (white arrow).

consistent with appendicitis. Meckel's may often be found incidentally during abdominal exploration or diagnosed in adults with persistent GI bleed without a source. Preoperative diagnosis of Meckel's diverticulum can be difficult. Plain films and ultrasound are not sensitive for the diagnosis. Computed tomography (CT) is only occasionally helpful. Technetium-99m pertechnetate imaging (Meckel scan) has high specificity for detection of associated ectopic gastric mucosa and a sensitivity of up to 83% for children presenting with lower GI bleeding (Figures 4.5a and 4.5b).

KEY POINTS

· Bloody stools in a neonate can be from a variety of etiologies such as benign anal fissures or milk protein allergy, or from more life-threatening etiologies such as volvulus, infectious colitis, or necrotizing enterocolitis (NEC).

· Other etiologies for bloody stools in older children include intussusception, usually diagnosed with ultrasound and treated

with contrast enema, or a Meckel's diverticulum, diagnosed with a technetium scintigraphy.
- NEC is most commonly seen in premature infants but must be excluded in infants presenting to the ED with bloody stools, especially in toxic infants requiring IV fluids and resuscitation.
- All NEC should be treated with IV fluids, bowel rest with gastric decompression and IV antibiotics, and surgical consultation.

TIPS FROM THE RADIOLOGIST

- An abdominal x-ray is the initial imaging modality of choice for the diagnosis of NEC.
- Pathognomonic features of NEC seen on x-ray include pneumatosis intestinalis (air within the bowel wall) or portal vein air. Pneumoperitoneum may occur from perforation.
- Ultrasound is also an emerging modality for diagnosis of NEC.

Further Reading

1. Bray-Aschenbrenner A, Feldenberg R, et al. Bloody stools in a 3-day-old term infant. *Pediatrics*. Sep 2017;140(3):e20170073. doi: 10.1543/peds,2017-0073.
2. Epelman M, Daneman A, Navarro OM, Morag I, Moore AM, Kim JH, Faingold R, Taylor G, Gerstle JT. Necrotizing enterocolitis: review of state-of-the-art imaging findings with pathologic correlation. *Radiographics*. 2007 Mar;27(2):285–305.
3. Kasivajjula H, Maheshwari A. Pathophysiology and current management of necrotizing enterocolitis. *Indian J Pediatr*. 2014 May;81(5):489–497. doi: 10.1007/s12098-014-1388-5. Epub 2014 Mar 22. PMID: 24652270.
4. Kim JH. Neonatal necrotizing enterocolitis. In: Post TW, ed. *UpToDate*. Waltham, MA: UpToDate. Accessed April 30, 2021.
5. Lin XK, Huang XZ, Bao XZ, Zheng N, Xia QZ, Chen CD. Clinical characteristics of Meckel diverticulum in children: a retrospective review of a 15-year single-center experience. *Medicine*. 2017 Aug;96(32):e7760. doi: 10.1097/MD.0000000000007760. PMID: 28796070; PMCID: PMC5556236.
6. Mandeville K, Chien M, Willyerd FA, et al. Intussusception: clinical presentations and imaging characteristics. *Pediatr Emerg Care*. 2012;28:842.
7. Medina LS, Applegate KE, Blackmore CC, eds. *Evidence-Based Imaging in Pediatrics: Optimizing Imaging in Pediatric Patient Care*. New York: Springer; 2010.
8. Sagar J, Kumar V, Shah DK. Meckel's diverticulum: a systematic review. *J R Soc Med*. 2006;99:501.

5 My Baby Won't Poop!

Yamini Jadcherla, Narendra Shet, and Maegan S. Reynolds

Case Study

A 35-day-old full-term healthy male presents to the emergency department for constipation. Pregnancy was uncomplicated, and the baby was born via spontaneous vaginal delivery with an uncomplicated postnatal course and was discharged home with mother after 24 hours. Mother states the baby did not have his first stool diaper until 3 days of life. It was non-bloody and dark green in color. Since birth, mother has been concerned about constipation, as he is only having one large explosive bowel movement every 5–7 days. He has had no fevers, and was tolerating breastfeeding, but in the past 24 hours he started having frequent nonbloody, nonbilious emesis and increased fussiness. At his pediatrician appointment today, he has only gained 3 ounces of weight since his 2-week visit. On evaluation he is afebrile, heart rate is 145 beats per minute, and oxygen saturation is 97% on room air. On exam the baby is fussy but consolable, has normal capillary refill and tone, but his abdomen is mildly distended.

What do you do now?

DIAGNOSIS/DISCUSSION

This infant's presentation is a concerning history for pathologic constipation and failure to thrive. Given that the patient is hemodynamically stable, emergent resuscitation is not required. Further workup is based on the degree of constipation and failure to thrive and the clinician's clinical concern for acute pathology.

Differential diagnosis for constipation in a neonate includes benign constipation, or more concerning pathology including Hirschsprung's disease, meconium ileus (often associated with cystic fibrosis), small left colon syndrome (common in infants of diabetic mothers), anorectal malformation, pseudo-obstruction, spinal cord anomalies (such as tethered cord), or hypothyroidism. Additionally, there is also a wide variation of what is considered "normal stools" in infants. Infants may stool several times per day or only once every 2–3 days. Breastfed infants typically have yellow, seedy stools many times per day. Formula-fed infants typically have thicker stools less frequently. Stool color can also vary, especially with formula-fed infants; the concerning colors are white (acholic stools are concerning for liver disease), or red/black (concerning for melena or hematochezia and gastrointestinal bleeding). Parents are often concerned about gas pain or constipation in infants. Due to weak abdominal muscles, infants often seem to be straining or grunting during bowel movements, which is not a sign of pathologic constipation. Concerning stool patterns are small hard pebble-like stools, straining with the development of anal fissures, or infrequent (i.e., weekly) large gushes of stools. Otherwise, there is a wide variety of normal stooling patterns, which can delay the diagnosis of a pathologic etiology. Infants rarely require medication for constipation; oral medications are not used, but rather parents can use an infrequent glycerin suppository or add a few ounces of pasteurized juice for infants over 1 month. In the Emergency Department (ED) if there are no other concerning features, such as delayed meconium passage, weight loss, dehydration, abnormal spine exam (i.e., sacral dimples, hair tufts, etc.), abdominal distension, the ED clinician can often refer an infant back to their pediatrician for ongoing constipation management.

However, if the infant's history is concerning for a pathologic etiology, further evaluation should be performed. Neonates typically lose weight after birth, but failure to return to their birth weight by 2 weeks of age, or weight loss of more than 10%, necessitates evaluation. Following 2 weeks of age, infants typically gain about 1 ounce per day, or about 0.5 pounds per week, though there is wide variability. However, weight loss is never normal, and poor weight gain is concerning. ED clinicians should review the growth chart of all infants with gastrointestinal complaints. An infant's failure to follow their growth curve necessitates further workup. In this case the infant has only gained 3 ounces in 3 weeks, thus falling off their growth curve. The additional described stooling pattern is concerning for Hirschsprung's disease and thus ED workup is indicated.

Hirschsprung's disease is also known as congenital aganglionic megacolon, which is caused by failed migration of colonic ganglion cells during fetal development. Typically, it affects the rectosigmoid; however, varying lengths of the colon and even small intestine can have aganglionic segments. Clinically, this results in colonic dysmotility, functional obstruction, constipation, progressive abdominal distention, and failure to thrive. This diagnosis is more common in boys and is associated with other conditions, most commonly linked with Trisomy 21, in up to 10% of patients, but also with visual and hearing impairment, congenital heart disease, and genitourinary abnormalities (most commonly hydronephrosis and renal dysplasia).

In the ED, the clinician should perform a rectal exam, assessing for anal fissures or tags externally and then perform an internal exam. Internal digital rectal exam is often notable for a tight anal sphincter and empty rectal vault. However, often immediately following, there is an explosive gush of gas and stools, also known as a "squirt sign." If there are signs of dehydration or failure to thrive, an IV should be placed and labs including electrolytes obtained. In assessing constipation, the initial imaging of choice is an abdominal x-ray. While a single supine x-ray can show increased colonic stool, at least two views, including a left lateral decubitus radiograph, should be obtained to assess for air-fluid levels.

The ED clinician should be able to recognize the varying stool patterns on infant abdominal radiographs. Normal stool patterns show gas throughout, including in the rectal vault (Figure 5.1). An infant with mild constipation may show increased stool throughout the colon (Figure 5.2). If there is a large stool ball in the sigmoid colon or rectal vault, this may

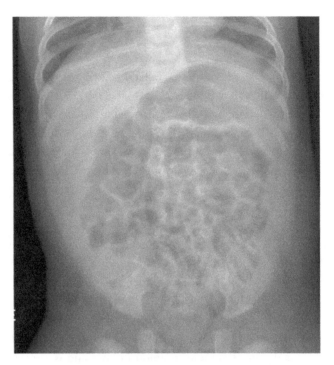

FIGURE 5.1. Normal AP radiograph of the abdomen in an infant.

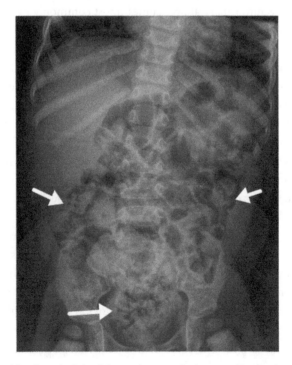

FIGURE 5.2. AP radiograph of the abdomen demonstrating large stool burden throughout the colon and rectum (white arrows) in a 1-year-old suspected of having constipation.

cause constipation with occasional watery stool, which is from overflow around the large stool ball. A large stool ball seen on x-ray or exam may require digital disimpaction or enema, especially in older infants or toddlers. Functional constipation can frequently be seen in toddlers undergoing potty-training. Additionally, urinary tract infections are common in older infants and toddlers with constipation, especially female patients.

Infants with Hirschsprung's disease may initially have a normal abdominal radiograph, but as they age and show clinical signs such as abdominal distension or failure to thrive, signs of bowel obstruction may be evident on x-ray. An abdominal radiography series can show progressive constipation, bowel distension, and eventually colonic distension with air-fluid levels (Figures 5.3a and 5.3b). In cases with delayed diagnosis or longer segments of aganglionic bowel wall, marked colon distension and dilation can be

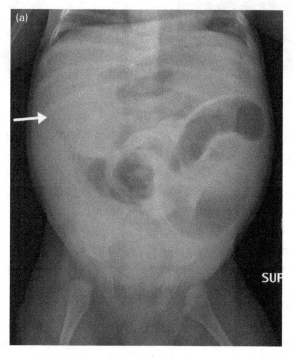

FIGURES 5.3a AND 5.3b. AP (a) and left lateral decubitus (b) radiographs of the abdomen in a 2-month-old demonstrate multiple dilated bowel loops with air-fluid levels in both small and large bowel noted on the decubitus view (b, white arrows). Note the presence of a large stool ball in the ascending colon (a, white arrow). Patient was eventually diagnosed with Hirschsprung's disease.

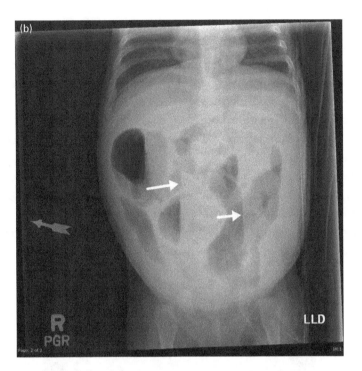

FIGURES 5.3a AND 5.3b. Continued

seen and may lead to perforation and pneumoperitoneum. If perforation is present, the infant will likely be ill-appearing and will need emergent resuscitation, IV antibiotics, and surgical intervention. If Hirschsprung's is suspected due to history or radiologic findings, additional radiographic studies can aid in diagnosis.

The most common additional imaging obtained is a fluoroscopy contrast enema. Bowel preparation is not needed prior to imaging. The contrast enema shows a segment of narrowing in the rectosigmoid colon with upstream proximal colonic distension. This transition zone from small caliber to dilation is pathognomonic for Hirschsprung's (Figures 5.4a and 5.4b). However, contrast enemas may also be normal up to the first 3 months of life, or may be normal indefinitely in those with total colonic involvement or ultra-short segment Hirschsprung's disease, thus delaying diagnosis even further. If there is high clinical suspicion but a transition zone is not detected on contrast enema, a post-evacuation abdominal radiograph may be obtained.

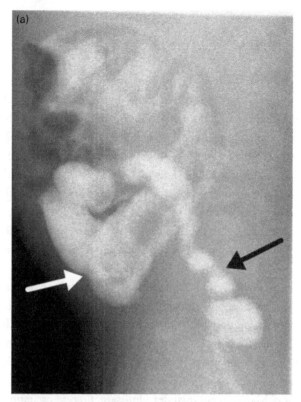

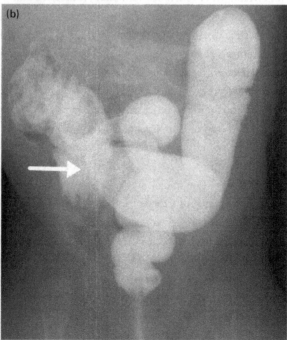

FIGURES 5.4a AND 5.4b. Lateral (a) and AP (b) images obtained during contrast enema in a patient with histopathologically confirmed Hirschsprung's disease. In Figure 5.4a, note the relatively narrow caliber of the rectum (black arrow) compared to the upstream sigmoid colon (white arrow), a characteristic finding in short segment Hirschsprung's disease. In Figure 5.4b, the degree of colonic dilatation relative to the rectum is again appreciated, with a suspected transition point (white arrow in b). The transition zone refers to the point where the normal bowel becomes aganglionic.

If a repeat abdominal x-ray 24 hours after the contrast enema shows retained contrast in the colon, this is highly suggestive of Hirschsprung's. Alternatively, anorectal manometry assessing the relaxation of the internal and external anal sphincter can aid in the diagnosis, especially for infants with ultra-short segment Hirschsprung's. However, a normal contrast enema or manometry cannot exclude the diagnosis of Hirschsprung's, and the diagnostic gold standard is rectal biopsy. A rectal biopsy 2 cm above the dentate line (physiologic aganglionosis is normal below the dentate line) showing aganglionosis confirms the diagnosis of Hirschsprung's. If high clinical concern remains despite a normal contrast enema, early referral to a pediatric surgeon is crucial.

It is also important to be mindful of complications associated with Hirschsprung's disease, both preoperatively and postoperatively, most commonly colonic perforation and enterocolitis. Enterocolitis has the highest incidence in the first 2 years after surgical repair but can present many years postoperatively. Patients with Hirschsprung-associated enterocolitis (HAEC) usually present with foul-smelling diarrhea, poor feeding, lethargy, and abdominal distention. Management includes admission, fluid resuscitation, rectal irrigation, and IV antibiotics (metronidazole or piperacillin-tazobactam).

Imaging of HAEC usually consists of radiographs, which often demonstrate bowel distention; however, patients with HAEC are at risk of perforation, in which case free air can be appreciated. Contrast enemas are contraindicated due to the risk of perforation.

In our case, given the high clinical concern for Hirschsprung's disease, secondary to delayed meconium passage and failure to thrive, a contrast enema was obtained which showed a transition zone confirming the diagnosis. The patient was admitted with a plan for operative repair with pediatric surgery. If the ED clinician has a high degree of clinical suspicion for Hirschsprung's by clinical history or initial abdominal radiographic imaging but an infant contrast enema is not available at your facility, referral to a tertiary pediatric hospital with advanced imaging and pediatric surgery is warranted. If the infant has mild constipation but a reassuring exam and abdominal x-rays, the pediatric surgery referral and/or contrast enema may be done on an outpatient non-emergent basis. However, if there are concerning features on ED imaging such as air-fluid levels, or the physical exam reveals significant abdominal tenderness or distension or failure to thrive, immediate transfer to pediatric tertiary care hospital may be indicated. Long term, most children do well following repair, but may be more prone to constipation, enterocolitis, or fecal incontinence.

KEY POINTS

- Constipation in an infant can be challenging, as it is often multifactorial, but clinicians should have a high degree of suspicion for Hirschsprung's disease if the patient presents with failure to pass meconium within the first 24 hours after delivery, infrequent but explosive bowel movements, progressive abdominal distention, or poor weight gain.
- Exam findings suggestive of Hirschsprung's disease include a tight anal sphincter with empty rectum and a positive "squirt sign" on rectal exam.
- Be mindful of complications associated with Hirschsprung's disease, such as colonic perforation and enterocolitis, which can even occur after surgical repair.

TIPS FROM THE RADIOLOGIST

- Abdominal radiographs in Hirschsprung's Disease typically show bowel distention, but in cases of delayed diagnosis or longer segment involvement, profound colonic distention may occur.
- Typical findings of Hirschsprung's disease on the contrast enema include a narrow segment of distal bowel with a transition to more proximal dilated bowel. The transition zone marks the site where the bowel becomes aganglionic.
- In HAEC, radiographs are typically the only imaging done, and are used to exclude bowel perforation. Contrast enemas are contraindicated due to the risk of bowel perforation.

Further Reading

1. Arshad A, Powell C, Tighe MP. Hirschsprung's disease. *BMJ*. 2012; 345:e5521.
2. Biggs WS, Dery WH. Evaluation and treatment of constipation in infants and children. *Am Fam Physician*. 2006;73(3):469–477.

3. Devos AS, Blickman JG, Blickman JG. *Radiological Imaging of the Digestive Tract in Infants and Children*. Cham: Springer Verlag; 2007.

4. Kessmann J. Hirschsprung's disease: diagnosis and management. *Am Fam Physician*. 2006;74(8):1319–1322.

5. Khan AR, Vujanic GM, Huddart S. The constipated child: how likely is Hirschsprung's disease? *Pediatr Surg Int*. 2003;19:439.

6. O'Donovan AN, Habra G, Somers S, Malone DE, Rees A, Winthrop AL. Diagnosis of Hirschsprung's disease. *AJR Am J Roentgenol*. 1996 Aug;167(2):517–520. doi: 10.2214/ajr.167.2.8686640. PMID: 8686640.

7. Swenson O. Hirschsprung's disease: a review. *Pediatrics*. 2002 May;109(5):914–918. doi: 10.1542/peds.109.5.914. PMID: 11986456.

8. Wesson DE, Lopez ME. Congenital aganglionic megacolon (Hirschsprung's disease). In: Post TW, ed., *UpToDate*. Waltham, MA: UpToDate. Accessed April 30, 2021.

6   Breathing through a Straw

Gina Pizzitola, David Teng, and Peter Assaad

Case Study

A 14-month-old male with a past medical history of reactive airway disease is brought back from triage with the chief complaint of respiratory distress. His parents report that he has had a runny nose for the past 2 days. He has also been drooling, which they had attributed to teething, although they note it seems worse today. The morning of presentation he developed a fever of 101.2°F, and all day he has been forcefully coughing. After dinner his parents noticed a "high-pitched" squeak as he was breathing, and, in a panic, rushed him to the Emergency Department (ED). On arrival to the ED he had a temperature of 101.5°F, his heart rate was 130 BPM, with a blood pressure of 118/83 mmHg. His respiratory rate was 35 breaths per minute, and he was actively crying. With every inspiration you hear a high-pitch sound best auscultated over his neck. There is otherwise no wheezing, rhonchi, or rales. His cardiac exam reveals tachycardia but no murmur. The rest of his exam is unremarkable.

What do you do now?

DISCUSSION

A child in respiratory distress can be terrifying both to parents and the clinician. The presence of stridor can prove to be a useful clinical clue in narrowing down your differential. When assessing a child with stridor, you will need to determine whether or not to pursue imaging. The recommended imaging selection will rest largely on your suspected diagnosis. Therefore, the following discussion is organized by etiology of stridor. In the setting of a "mixed picture," it may be necessary to obtain multiple images to rule out one etiology and confirm another.

Suspected Croup

Croup, also known as laryngotracheomalacia, is the most common cause of inspiratory stridor in children. It is commonly preceded by a runny nose, is most identifiable by a cough often described as "barking" (like a dog or a seal), and frequently improves when the parents take the child outdoors into the winter cold. Croup usually affects children between 6 months and 3 years of age. With such a distinct symptom profile, croup is a clinical diagnosis, and imaging is generally not required to diagnose it. However, there are some scenarios in which imaging can be helpful, such as when there is concomitant concern for aspiration of a foreign body. For example, in the case presented, the child's progression appears infectious in the setting of a fever and rhinorrhea; however, the stridor began after dinner, thus elevating the possibility that the child had aspirated a piece of food. In such a situation, you may begin by obtaining posteroanterior (PA) and lateral images of the neck and/or chest.

Classically, a PA plain film in croup will reveal a "steeple sign." As depicted in Figure 6.1, this sign is the result of progressive narrowing of the trachea. This narrowing results in the development of stridor. A lateral neck x-ray may reveal tracheal narrowing, but also should be evaluated for signs of epiglottitis. In croup the epiglottis will be normal in appearance (Figure 6.2).

As stated before, croup is a clinical diagnosis, and you likely will initially forgo imaging if your suspicion for croup is high. If you treat with racemic epinephrine and the stridor fails to improve, you should revisit your differential and consider imaging for another diagnosis, such as foreign body, which you would not expect to respond to medical treatments.

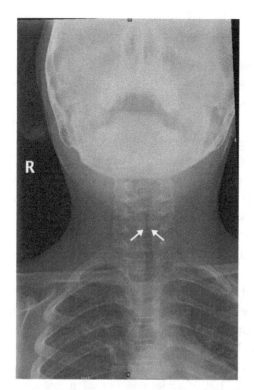

FIGURE 6.1. PA neck x-ray shows classic steeple sign (arrows) created by narrowing of the trachea in croup.

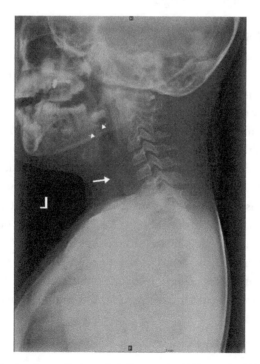

FIGURE 6.2. Lateral neck x-ray displays subglottic narrowing (thick arrow), which can cause stridor heard in croup. Normal epiglottis (thin arrows) is noted.

Suspected Foreign Body

Aspiration of a foreign body that lands in the upper airway (pharynx, larynx, trachea) or in the upper esophagus may result in stridor. A foreign body in the upper airway creates stridor when it only partially obstructs airflow, thereby creating a narrower than normal area where air passes through. As air quickly travels through this narrow space, it creates the high-pitch sound of stridor. A foreign body in the upper esophagus creates the same effect by pushing on the wall of the esophagus and compressing the trachea, again decreasing the area through which air passes.

When there is concern for a foreign body, you should consider PA and lateral neck plain films. In order to most accurately interpret the film, it is important to know if the object that may have been aspirated is radiopaque. Ideally you will be able to see the object on x-ray; however, if the object is not radiopaque, a "negative" x-ray will not help you eliminate the possibility of foreign body aspiration. In such a case you may need to pursue bronchoscopy. Furthermore, we want to emphasize that the presence of stridor suggests the foreign body is in a location that would impinge on the upper airway. The lack of stridor does not mean absence of a foreign body, but rather suggests that if there is a foreign body, it has moved beyond the upper airway or upper esophagus.

Suspected Epiglottitis

In a world where most children are vaccinated against haemophilus influenza B (HiB), epiglottitis is a rare diagnosis. Nevertheless, epiglottitis can be caused by infectious as well as noninfectious etiologies, and therefore, it must remain on your differential for the child with stridor.[1]

As with croup, radiologic imaging is not required for diagnosis of epiglottitis, although it may be helpful in conjunction with the clinical exam. When deciding to obtain imaging for epiglottitis, it is of utmost importance to consider the stability of the child and his or her potential for decompensation. Children with true epiglottitis are at risk for rapid deterioration secondary to airway obstruction. This may be precipitated by emotional distress (crying) or repositioning of the patient (from tripod to supine) or laryngospasm. You should obtain imaging when your suspicion for the diagnosis is high, but the child is stable and calm without immediate or imminent need for direct visualization and/or intubation. Ideally, imaging should be obtained in the ED, but if necessary to move the child to radiology it is essential that appropriate airway equipment and personnel accompany the child.

On a lateral neck x-ray of a child with epiglottitis, you will expect to see the "thumb sign," which is created by an inflamed swollen epiglottis (Figure 6.3). Swollen aryepiglottic folds may also be observed.

Suspected Retropharyngeal Abscess

In a child that is drooling and febrile, the presence of a retropharyngeal abscess (RPA) should be considered. RPAs are most commonly seen in children less than 4 years old. The most commonly implicated bacteria is Group A beta-hemolytic strep. The selection of imaging modality should depend on the level of suspicion as well as the severity of presentation. In a stable child with low likelihood of an RPA, you may start with a lateral neck x-ray.

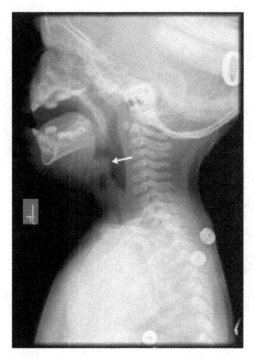

FIGURE 6.3. The lateral neck x-ray shows the "thumb sign," caused by an inflamed swollen epiglottis (arrow), as well as swollen aryepiglottic folds.

The lateral neck x-ray of a child with a suspected RPA should be evaluated for prevertebral widening. Positioning is critical. The image needs to be a true lateral shot obtained with the head in "normal extension" while the patient is inspiring to avoid false positives. Please note that an image obtained while the child is crying may also result in a false positive. Cellulitis or abscess in the retropharyngeal space will cause prevertebral widening on imaging. An image is considered positive for RPA if the width of the prevertebral soft tissue is larger than expected. The expected normal width varies based on vertebral level. From C1 to C4, the upper limit of normal would be about equal to one-half the width of a vertebral body. From C5 to C7, the upper limit of normal would be about equal to the width of one vertebral body.

While a lateral neck x-ray can help you screen for an RPA (Figure 6.4), computed tomography (CT) of the neck with contrast will

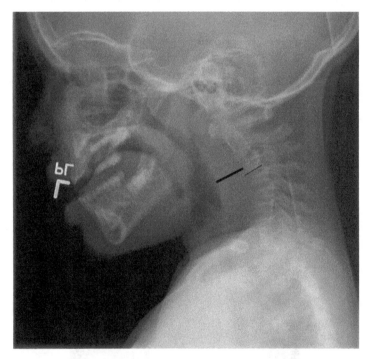

FIGURE 6.4. The lateral neck x-ray shows prevertebral widening (thick black line), which is consistent with a retropharyngeal abscess. Compare the prevertebral space thickness to the much smaller vertebral body size of C3 (thin black line).

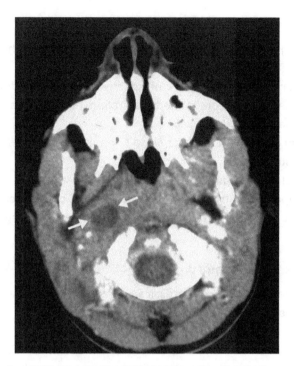

FIGURE 6.5. An axial CT slice below the skull base shows a rim enhancing abscess (arrows) in the right retropharyngeal space.

offer you better characterization of the infected area (Figure 6.5), including presence of abscess versus cellulitis. While more detailed imaging will be beneficial in diagnosing an RPA, it has the additional benefit of providing guidance for surgical treatment (i.e., mapping out vasculature).

The child in the described case would benefit from a plain film. His history of upper respiratory symptoms and forceful cough makes croup the most likely diagnosis; however, the development of stridor after dinner raises the possibility of foreign body aspiration. As such, the child received a plain film, which showed a steeple sign, confirming the diagnosis of croup. The child received a single epinephrine aerosol, a dose of dexamethasone, and was discharged without complication after about 4 hours.

- Imaging is not always necessary in croup; however, if the patient fails to respond to medical management, x-rays may help support the diagnosis while decreasing suspicion for other etiologies such as foreign body aspiration, epiglottitis, and retropharyngeal abscesses.
- Foreign objects in the upper airway or upper esophagus may cause stridor.
- Be careful not to put patients with epiglottitis at further risk of decompensation by pursuing images outside of the department without appropriate medical supervision and monitoring.

- A PA chest x-ray in croup classically reveals the "steeple sign."
- Lateral soft tissue neck x-ray in epiglottitis classically reveals the "thumb sign."
- Plain films can be a good initial study to evaluate for RPA.
- CT scan is better at characterizing abscess versus cellulitis in an RPA, with the added benefit of vascular mapping in preparation for surgical intervention.

Further Reading

1. Lai S-H, Wong K-S, Liao S-L, Chou Y-H. Non-infectious epiglottitis in children: two cases report. *Int J Pediatr Otorhinolaryngol*. 2000;55(1):57–60. ISSN 0165-5876. https://doi.org/10.1016/S0165-5876(00)00376-1.
2. Zitelli BJ, McIntire S, Nowalk AJ. *Atlas of Pediatric Physical Diagnosis*. 7th ed. Philadelphia: Elsevier; 2017.

7   Drooling, Drooling, Drooling All the Way Home

Brooke Lampl, Nkeiruka Orajiaka, and Meika Eby

Case Presentation

A previously healthy 14-month-old male presents to the emergency room with the acute onset of a choking episode and drooling that started 4 hours ago.

He was playing at home unsupervised when his mother suddenly heard him coughing intermittently. Mother states he was standing by a drawer where old items were stored. His face appeared red. He has refused feeds since then. He has had no fever, runny nose, diarrhea, or trouble breathing.

Past medical history is unremarkable. He was the full-term product of an uncomplicated pregnancy and delivery. His immunizations are up to date.

His temperature is 98.7°F, heart rate 110 BPM, respiratory rate 30 BPM, and blood pressure 90/60mmHg. He appears uncomfortable, leaning forward and drooling intermittently. He is not in respiratory distress. His oral exam shows no objects or lesions. His abdominal exam and extremities are normal.

What do you do now?

DISCUSSION

Given the child's age and acute onset of cough, vomiting, and food refusal, ingestion of a foreign body was suspected. The child was assigned a nil by mouth status and urgent imaging was obtained.

Radiographs are the primary imaging modality used in the evaluation of suspected ingested foreign bodies. In order to determine the location of a radiopaque foreign body, anteroposterior (AP) and lateral views of the neck, chest, and/or abdomen may be obtained depending on the clinical picture. Esophageal foreign bodies most commonly become lodged at the thoracic inlet or aortic arch and less frequently at the lower esophageal sphincter. In addition to location, radiographs provide information regarding the size, shape, and number of foreign bodies, which can aid in clinical management.

In the United States, the most common pediatric foreign bodies ingested are coins, followed by a variety of other objects, including toys, sharp objects, and batteries. Magnets, button batteries, and sharp objects require special attention as they are associated with increased morbidity.

Button batteries will be discussed in detail in Chapter 8. In the event that radiographs are negative and a foreign body is still suspected, sub-specialty consultation is indicated. Non-radiopaque foreign bodies may include glass, fish bones, plastic toys, and aluminum pull-tabs, as well as more recently crystal gel balls. Fluoroscopy with oral contrast (esophogram) may outline a non-radiopaque foreign body in the esophagus. In some instances, computed tomography (CT) may be helpful in the evaluation of some non-radiopaque foreign bodies, particularly in the airway (American College of Radiology practice guidelines for pediatric CT), or in the evaluation of complications associated with foreign bodies, such as perforation, inflammatory mass, and tracheoesophageal or esophageal-aortic fistula.

Coins

Coins in the esophagus typically appear *en face* (circular) on AP films (Figure 7.1a) and on their side (thinner oval/slit like) on lateral films (Figure 7.1b), whereas when in the trachea, coins will appear *en face* on the lateral view.

Up to 25% of coins will spontaneously pass within 8–16 hours of ingestion. Successful passage depends on the location of the coin, the age of the

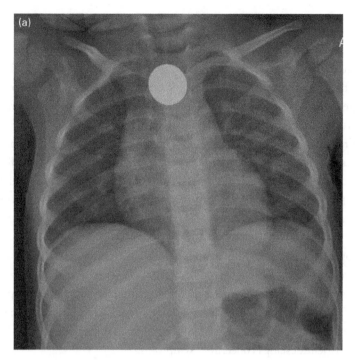

FIGURE 7.1a. Frontal radiograph of the chest with a round foreign body, compatible with a coin, at the thoracic inlet.

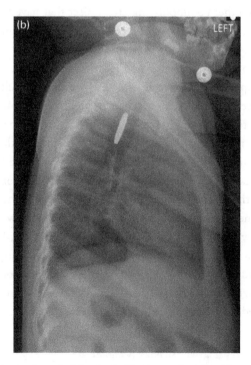

FIGURE 7.1b. Lateral radiograph of the chest with coin seen in profile at the upper mediastinum, confirming esophageal location.

child, and the size of the coin. Most foreign bodies in the upper or mid-esophagus will not pass, whereas lower esophageal coins tend to advance into the stomach and pass without incident. In children less than 5 years of age, coins larger than 23.5 mm are also less likely to advance beyond the pylorus.

Urgent removal is indicated for esophageal coins in acutely symptomatic distressed patients, such as those with respiratory distress or inability to maintain secretions. Otherwise, if the coin is in the esophagus (regardless of symptoms), removal within 24 hours is recommended if it has not otherwise spontaneously passed on repeat imaging. If the coin is in the stomach and the patient is asymptomatic or does not have severe symptoms, expectant management at home with straining stools and strict return precautions is recommended, with repeat films every 1–2 weeks to ensure passage. Endoscopic removal is recommended for gastric coins that have not passed after 2–4 weeks. For coins that have passed beyond the stomach, the same home expectant management is recommended, as removal is indicated only if the patient develops concerning symptoms.

Magnets

Magnets are another commonly ingested object that have been associated with significant morbidity and even mortality, with complications including bowel ischemia/necrosis, perforation, fistula, obstruction, and peritonitis. It is important to note the number and location of magnets. There is a risk of bowel entrapment and necrosis with the ingestion of multiple magnets, as they become attracted to each other through the gastrointestinal tract. Due to magnetic attraction, it can be difficult to determine the number of magnets if the magnets are stacked or attracted to one another. If this is of concern, magnification views, fluoroscopy, or CT may be helpful. Serial radiographs may also be helpful in magnet ingestion in order to ensure movement of the magnets throughout the gastrointestinal tract; a static location of magnets on sequential films raises concern for bowel entrapment.

For both symptomatic and asymptomatic patients with multiple (≥ 2) magnets or a magnet plus another metallic foreign body, urgent removal is indicated if endoscopy can be utilized (either esophagogastroduodenoscopy or colonoscopy). This may be performed by a pediatric gastrointestinal specialist or a pediatric surgeon depending on the institution. For multiple magnets between the duodenal-jejunal junction and the terminal ileum, management is controversial and should be discussed with both pediatric gastroenterology and pediatric surgery if available. If there is a single magnet only, consultation with a pediatric gastroenterologist is recommended as management options include removal or outpatient serial x-rays.

Sharp Objects

Sharp objects such as nails, pins/tacks, toothpicks, and bones also require special consideration, with the latter two objects being the highest risk for perforation and the most common to require surgical removal (Figure 7.2). Though most will pass without incident, complications include perforation/

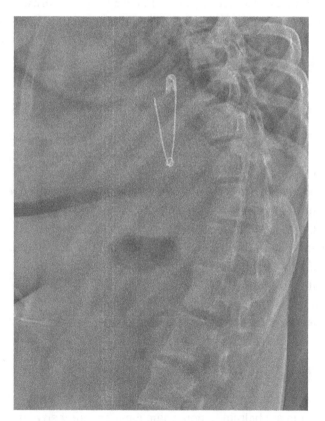

FIGURE 7.2. Lateral view of the chest and abdomen demonstrates an open safety pin lodged in the lower esophagus at the gastroesophageal junction. This was subsequently removed by endoscopy during which a perforation in the esophageal wall was detected.

fistula, extraluminal migration, infection/abscess, organ penetration, arterial rupture, aortoesophageal fistula, and death.

As previously mentioned, glass, fish bones, and plastic toys may not be seen on plain films, and wood is completely radiolucent. Management is based on symptoms, location, and the type of object. Sharp objects in the esophagus are very high risk and require emergent removal.

Case Conclusion

Our patient presented with symptoms suggestive of an acute foreign body ingestion. Though he initially presented with choking, our patient had a stable respiratory exam besides drooling intermittently. Foreign body radiographs showed a circular object without a halo in the distal esophagus. The foreign body team was consulted and due to continued symptoms of drooling and vomiting, our patient was taken to the operating room for endoscopic removal of a swallowed coin.

KEY POINTS

- Patients presenting with swallowed foreign bodies may be asymptomatic or have various, nonspecific symptoms, requiring a high index of suspicion.
- Button batteries, multiple magnets, and sharp objects have higher risk of morbidity and mortality.
- The European Society for Pediatric Gastroenterology, Hepatology, and Nutrition (ESPGHAN) and the North American Society for Pediatric Gastroenterology, Hepatology, and Nutrition (NASPHGHAN) have created management guidelines for ingested foreign bodies.
- The National Capital Poison Center has a hotline (202-625-3333).

TIPS FROM THE RADIOLOGIST

- Frontal and lateral radiographs of the neck, chest, and/or abdomen are helpful to determine location, number, and characteristics of the foreign body.

- If radiographs are negative for radiopaque foreign body and one is still suspected, additional imaging, including decubitus radiographs of the chest, may be helpful to evaluate for air trapping from a non-radiopaque foreign body.
- CT can be useful for assessing complications associated with foreign bodies.

Further Reading

1. Kramer RE, Lerner DG, Lin T, et al. Management of ingested foreign bodies in children: a clinical report of the NASPGHAN Endoscopy Committee. *J Pediatr Gastroenterol Nutr.* 2015;60(4):562–574. doi: 10.1097/MPG.0000000000000729.
2. Orsagh-Yentis D, McAdams RJ, Roberts KJ, McKenzie LB. Foreign-body ingestions of young children treated in US emergency departments: 1995–2015. *Pediatrics.* 2019;143(5):e20181988. doi: 10.1542/peds.2018-1988.
3. Louie MC, Bradin S. Foreign body ingestion and aspiration. *Pediatr Rev.* 2009;30(8):295–301. doi: 10.1542/pir.30-8-295.
4. Chung S, Forte V, Campisi P. A review of pediatric foreign body ingestion and management. *Clin Pediatr Emerg Med.* 2010;11(3):225–230.
5. Guelfguat M, Kaplinskiy V, Reddy SH, DiPoce J. Clinical guidelines for imaging and reporting ingested foreign bodies. *Am J Roentgenol.* 2014;203(1):37–53.
6. Laya BF, Restrepo R, Lee EY. Practical imaging evaluation of foreign bodies in children: an update. *Radiol Clin.* 2017;55(4):845–867.
7. Waltzman ML, Baskin M, Wypij D, Mooney D, Jones D, Fleisher G. A randomized clinical trial of the management of esophageal coins in children. *Pediatrics.* 2005;116(3):614–619.
8. Kay M, Wyllie R. Pediatric foreign bodies and their management. *Curr Gastroenterol Rep.* 2005;7(3):212–218.
9. Pugmire BS, Lin TK, Pentiuk S, de Alarcon A, Hart CK, Trout AT. Imaging button battery ingestions and insertions in children: a 15-year single-center review. *Pediatr Radiol.* 2017;47(2):178–185.
10. Eggli KD, Potter BM, Garcia V, Altman RP, Breckbill DL. Delayed diagnosis of esophageal perforation by aluminum foreign bodies. *Pediatr Radiol.* 1986;16(6):511–513.

8 Burn, Baby, Burn

Cory Gotowka, Ailish Coblentz, and Michael Stoner

Case Report

A previously healthy 18-month-old male was seen in his local urgent care for the acute onset of food aversion, agitation, and coughing spells starting earlier today. The mother reports no history of stridor, wheezing, or respiratory distress. His mother states that he had eaten his breakfast in typical fashion and later he began to cough up his morning snack, around 10:30 am. His parents brought him to a local pediatric urgent care around 11:45am, where a posteroanterior chest x-ray showed a 24mm circular, metallic foreign body spanning his second and third thoracic vertebrae (Figure 8.1). He was immediately transported to a pediatric Emergency Department (ED).

When he arrived at the ED at 1:45pm, he was uncomfortable, coughing occasionally, and had intermittent gagging episodes with anterior-leaning positioning.

What do you do now?

DIAGNOSIS

In this case, the patient had no preceding signs of illness and no trauma. Aside from a cough and occasional gag, this child was without other respiratory symptoms, and was having an aversion to food, which likely represents an esophageal obstruction. Given the sudden onset, one must consider food bolus or foreign body ingestion causing an obstruction. It is especially important to ask parents and take note of all of the possibilities that could have been ingested: magnets, fishbones, chicken bones, batteries, coins, etc., as the treatment and urgency rely on identification first and foremost. Therefore, after addressing any airway, breathing or circulation issues, the next step should be diagnostic.

Although there was not a witnessed ingestion of a foreign body, this must remain high on the differential diagnosis. In our case, he was immediately sent for a chest x-ray, which suggested that a radio-opaque foreign body was in his proximal esophagus (Figures 8.1 and 8.2). In any other instance without radiographic confirmation of foreign body ingestion, if there is still a high index of suspicion, then a swallow study or a direct endoscopy should be considered. The location of the foreign body in this case correlates clinically, given his food aversion and respiratory stability.

The radiologist calls you, to make you aware of a double-density border (also known as a halo sign and the step-off sign), very suggestive for a button battery (BB). The radiologist notes that there are standard sizes for all button batteries and coins for radiographic comparison, and this 24mm radio-opaque foreign body was consistent with a button battery. The radiologist was sure to indicate the smaller (negative pole/anode) side of the BB and area of contact. The ingestion of a noncaustic foreign body like a coin is treated very differently than a button battery ingestion. Rarely two stacked coins (a nickel and a dime) stuck together can show a double-density border or a halo sign as well.

The mother of the child did not witness him ingest anything, and there was no evidence of a battery-powered toy, remote, or a watch that had been taken apart. The timeline suggests that this ingestion may have occurred sometime between his breakfast at 07:00 am and his mid-morning snack at 10:00 am, and it is now 2:45 pm.

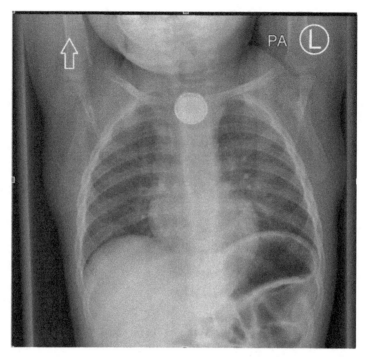

FIGURE 8.1. Posteroanterior chest radiograph of an 18-month-old child demonstrating a 24mm metallic foreign body in-line with the esophagus, spanning the second to third vertebrae. The foreign body has two visible rings, which correspond to the "halo sign," consistent with a button battery. Note the peripheral irregularity of the battery that is compatible with corrosion.

TREATMENT

It has been, at most, eight hours since the ingestion, and the longer the BB is in the esophagus, the more damage it can do. The battery needs to be removed, but since it is suspected that the ingestion was less than 12 hours prior, the patient should receive 10 mL of oral honey or sucralfate every 10 minutes until you can remove it.[1,2] Honey should not be given to children < 1 year of age but is otherwise readily available prehospital. Once in the ED, switch to sucralfate until the child can get to the endoscopy suite. Sucralfate and honey can coat the BB and prevent further necrotic injury. Of note, this is a temporizing strategy and should not delay getting the patient to the endoscopy suite.

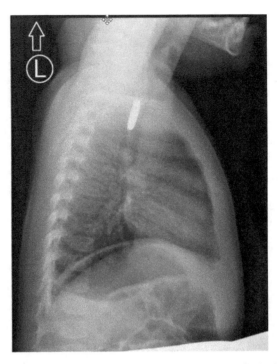

FIGURE 8.2. Lateral chest radiograph demonstrating that the radiopaque foreign body is in the proximal esophagus at the level of the thoracic inlet. The foreign body is flat and has a "step-off sign" and the direction of the smaller pole is posterior, which is diagnostic for a button battery ingestion. Note the peripheral irregularity of the battery that is compatible with corrosion.

Next the patient needs someone comfortable with both endoscopy and extraction. Direct-visualization via endoscope is much preferred to other modes of retrieval, which might include balloon catheter or magnet retrieval. Direct visualization allows you to quantify the extent, depth, and location of mucosal injury. In most academic centers, there are three options: a general or pediatric surgeon, an otolaryngologist, or a gastroenterologist, though this is not an all-inclusive list. Removal is considered an emergency, and should not be postponed for any reason, including lack of NPO status. In our case, given the patient's clinical stability, we called Pediatric General Surgery to assess the chest radiographs and give their recommendations.

In the interim, should you obtain other labs? Blood counts might be a late indicator of hemorrhage if a perforation is present; however, his blood pressure and other vital signs were stable, so that is unlikely. A blood gas might help determine the extent of respiratory involvement, but given the paucity of respiratory symptoms in our patient, it was not indicated. He was made NPO, a peripheral IV was placed, maintenance rate of IV fluids was started, and an IV proton pump inhibitor was started while he was being transported to the endoscopy suite.

Some institutions treat patients with oral acidic cocktails and/or liquid vitamin C washes to reduce damage and to try to neutralize the alkalotic microenvironment, especially if there is a prolonged transit to a different hospital for removal. This is not the national standard of care. You should never induce vomiting or give a laxative. Once the patient is undergoing endoscopy, direct visualization has been obtained and has confirmed that a perforation is not present, the area is to be irrigated with 0.25% sterile acetic acid to neutralize the alkaline environment. This has been shown to improve outcomes and prevent alkaline induced liquefactive necrosis.[2,3]

DISCUSSION

Foreign body ingestion (FBI) is a common occurrence in the pediatric patient.[4] When there is a high suspicion for an ingested foreign body, a rapid diagnosis is imperative. Identification of the foreign body is critical, as a coin FBI is treated differently than a button battery ingestion (BBI). If it is the latter, timing is one of the greatest prognostic indicators for complications and lethality.[5] Button batteries are the second most frequently ingested foreign bodies, second to coins.[5] Unfortunately, the incidence of BBI continues to rise, with an average of 3,500 annually in the United States.[6] National Electronic Injury Surveillance System has shown the absolute number of ED visits for battery-related injury has more than doubled from 1990 to 2009,[7] with 63% occurring in children younger than 6 years of age.[8] In addition to the increase in incidence, the rate of significant complications and death resulting from BBI has increased nearly sevenfold,[9] with the majority of serious outcomes and fatalities occurring in children between the ages of 1 and 3 years. In children younger than 6 years old who ingest a 20mm BB (or larger), serious or fatal outcomes occur 12.6% of the time.[10] This increased morbidity and mortality are hypothesized to be due to the larger diameter and more powerful lithium ion batteries being more commonly available in household items and independently around the house.

PATHOPHYSIOLOGY

The physiology of the caustic mucosal-injury caused by a BB occurs when the moisture of the digestive tract mucosa bridges the positive and negative terminals of the battery, thus closing the circuit and allowing current to flow into the local tissue. Electrical current from the battery results in the generation of hydroxide radicals, which rapidly raises the pH of the microenvironment, leading to alkalotic burns and subsequent liquefactive necrosis.[11] This necrosis can weaken the mucosa in a short period of time and has been demonstrated to start within 15 minutes of contact.[12] The anode (smaller pole) of the BB is responsible for the majority of the more significant burns. Battery retention time may be one of the most important influencing factors for the formation of one of the more fatal complications, an esophageal fistula. The risk of severe complications such as tracheoesophageal fistula, esophageal perforation, and aortic hemorrhage significantly increases if the retention time is greater than 24 hours.[5]

Even with batteries that have been ingested after being used, significant injury may still be possible.[13] This demonstrates the power of the newer lithium batteries, which have a much longer shelf life than traditional alkaline batteries, and when they are no longer useful to power the electronic device, they still have some residual electrical power.[9] The majority of children who suffer from BBI obtain them from household items such as remote controls, games or toys, calculators, and watches.[10]

PRESENTING SYMPTOMS

The most common presenting symptoms of a child with a BBI include vomiting, fever, anorexia, cough, difficulty managing secretions, salivation, and breathing difficulties (dyspnea, dysphagia, stridor).[1] Infants less than 1 year old may also present with anorexia, irritability, or tarry stools, while children older than 5 years old may present with abdominal pain or chest pain.[5] These presenting symptoms can be very nonspecific, and therefore can be easily misdiagnosed as a viral illness or other nonspecific etiology.[14]

A delay in diagnosis and removal can increase the risk of serious outcomes, so a high clinical index of suspicion is essential to reduce morbidity and mortality. When there is a high clinical suspicion (even in the absence of a radiographic finding), patients can also go straight to direct visualization for removal via bronchoscopy or esophagoscopy.

COMPLICATIONS

Devastating complications are more likely to occur if the local pH is not neutralized upon diagnosis and/or removal, and therefore can cause continued caustic alkalotic injury. Button batteries most commonly lodge in the stenosis of esophagus around which the trachea, mediastinum, and great vessels exist.[5] Complications that can occur from ingestion include tracheoesophageal fistula, aortoesophageal fistula, esophageal perforation which could lead to mediastinitis, esophageal strictures, vocal cord paralysis with subsequent aspiration, as well as battery aspiration into the bronchial tree. The esophagus is the most affected organ, and aortoesophageal fistula is the most feared complication, as vascular involvement is often fatal.[15] Of the 65 fatal BBIs since 1977, 26 of the deaths were caused by aortoesophageal fistulas (40%), and 12 of the deaths were caused by tracheoesophageal fistulas (18%), and this is due to the risk of progression to rapid and catastrophic hemorrhage.[14, 15] Any child with a history of recently removed BB presenting with hematemesis or coffee-ground emesis should be considered to have aortoesophageal fistula until proven otherwise.

If there is any concern for a complication, then computed tomography (CT) would be the imaging modality of choice. CT is also occasionally used for better delineation/anatomic understanding prior to an interventional procedure, providing better delineation of a foreign body, infection/abscess, or area of injury. In the case of an aortoesophageal fistula, CT scan of the chest must be performed to associate the proximity of the fistula to essential anatomic organs that could lead to catastrophic hemorrhage (aortic arch, azygos vein) (Figure 8.3).

It has also been reported that children with minimal mucosal injury upon removal of button battery may present days to weeks later with progressive damage.[5] The timing of associated morbidity from BB exposure can be unpredictable, in part because the majority of BBI are not witnessed.

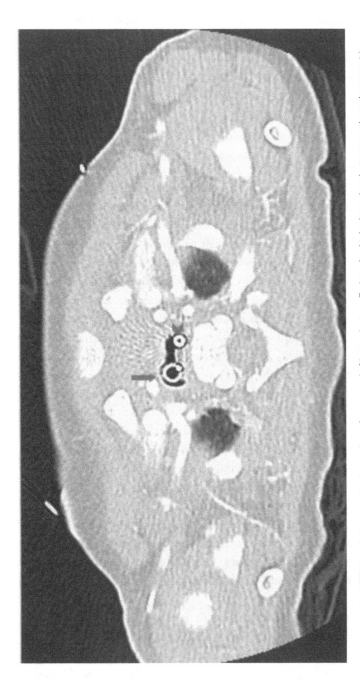

FIGURE 8.3. Axial CT chest in lung window in a patient after removal of button battery. Endotracheal tube (arrow) and a transesophageal nasogastric tube (arrowhead) have been placed. A large tracheoesophageal fistula is seen connecting the two lumens. This is secondary to severe caustic injury.

More than 50% of serious outcomes due to BBI occur after unwitnessed ingestions, in which case there is likely a delay in recognition and diagnosis.[9,10] This emphasizes the necessity for pediatric ED providers to act quickly in both the diagnosis and the initiation of the team for removal of the foreign body.

Negative prognostic indicators for BBI include: the age of the patient, size of the battery, timing of ingestion, and the current location of the battery. These encompass the most important risk factors for predicting severe injury, necessitating the highest level of concern: esophageal impaction at the level of the aortic arch, age less than 5 years, battery size of 20mm or greater, and prolonged time of impaction.[9] Despite a reassuring esophogram and clinical stability 5 days after ingestion, devastating hemorrhage from esophageal erosion secondary to BBI can unexpectedly occur weeks out from the initial ingestion.[5] Any child who is over 4 weeks out from BB removal presenting with food refusal should be considered to have a stricture until proven otherwise.

CASE RESOLUTION

Within the hour, our patient had an endoscopy performed by the general surgery team. A 24mm lithium button battery was removed using forceps with endoscopic guidance. The battery's positive side read "+ CR2477 Lithium Battery 3V." The esophagus was irrigated with 100 mL of 0.25% sterile acetic acid to help neutralize the area. The endoscopist obtained images which showed moderate mucosal edema with erosive necrosis and a central area of eschar. There was no evidence of frank blood or hemorrhage.

After awakening from sedation, the patient was admitted to the hospital for observation. Given his moderate edema, evidence of eschar, and with a posterior esophageal burn near the aortic arch, he was admitted to the Pediatric Intensive Care Unit (PICU).

Our patient was started on broad spectrum antibiotics, and a nasogastric (NG) tube was placed for gastric decompression. It has been shown that decompression of the stomach contents has reduced esophageal mucosal injury and subsequently morbidity in BBIs, and proton pump inhibitors are used in 75% of BBIs. After 36 hours of continued stability, his NG tube was transitioned to provide enteral NG feeds, which were up-titrated as his IVF was sequentially weaned. Lateral esophogram with barium was performed on hospital day 4, which showed no evidence of esophageal perforation, and his NG tube was removed. In the subsequent days his diet was advanced from clear liquids to a soft diet. He was discharged on hospital day 7 without further complication. He had a repeat barium esophogram and follow-up with ENT 30 days post ingestion.

SPECIAL CONSIDERATIONS

Are there any indications to not remove? Yes! Current AAP button battery ingestion guidelines recommend that in the case of a child older than 12 years old without prior history of esophageal disease, who ingests just one battery that is less than 12mm (either via radiography or with historical certainty), and the patient is asymptomatic, then that child can be monitored at home while monitoring for battery passage in stool.[1] Radiographs should be reconsidered if there is no passage within two weeks.[1] There is almost no utility in ultrasonography unless wanting to assess the location of the foreign body, for instance to assess if it has surpassed the ileo-cecal valve. This may be more important if co-ingestion occurred with a magnet. Hearing aid batteries can almost always be considered to be smaller than 12mm. In a case where removal is not recommended, parents should know the red flag symptoms for return.

What do I do if the battery is in the stomach?

The management of asymptomatic patients with batteries beyond the esophagus is still up for clinical consideration and debate. In 2015, the North American Society for Pediatric Gastroenterology, Hepatology and Nutrition Endoscope (NASPHGHAN) Committee proposed that in children with a gastric button battery and the following factors, such as 5 years older or above, short duration of ingestion (<2 hours), size of the battery <20 mm, absence of clinical symptoms, observation may be used.[17] Consistent with American Society for Gastrointestinal Endoscopy guidelines, larger batteries (≥20 mm) in the stomach should be checked by radiograph and removed if in place after >48 hours.

The National Capital Poison Control Center's button battery triage and treatment guideline suggests that if there is no co-ingestion with a magnet, the battery is less than 15mm, the child is older than 6 years old, then observation alone is warranted. However, practitioners should be aware that even after passage of the battery to the stomach, necrosis can continue as the battery passes through the gastrointestinal tract.[5] If a patient at any point becomes symptomatic, removal is always indicated regardless of battery positioning.[1]

KEY POINTS

- As soon as possible, initiate the sequence for removing the BB. Get the proper personnel and location of endoscopic intervention (surgeon vs. otolaryngologist vs. gastroenterologist, and bedside vs. operating room vs. endoscopy suite), and assess if sedation is necessary.
- If ingestion occurred less than 12 hours prior, the patient should receive 10 mL of oral honey (>1 year of age), or sucralfate. Both can be readministered every 10 minutes but should not delay removal.
- Removal of the BB ASAP with endoscopic imaging immediately post removal.

  Rinsing with acidic solution under endoscopy can effectively improve the prognosis. NPO, NG tube placement, and subsequent gastrointestinal decompression, IVF, as well as IV proton pump inhibitors, can be used to prevent the regurgitation of gastric juice, thus protecting the friable digestive mucosa

---

TIPS FROM THE RADIOLOGIST

- A child presenting to the ED with symptoms consistent with a foreign body should have both anteroposterior and lateral radiographs of the chest to locate and diagnose BBI.
- A double-density border (also known as a halo sign and the step-off sign), is extremely suggestive for a BB.
- Note the orientation of the slightly smaller negative pole (anode) as the likely side of mucosal injury.
- There are standard sizes for all BBs and coins for radiographic comparison.

- Rarely two stacked coins (a nickel and a dime) stuck together can show a double-density border or a halo sign as well.
- CT can be used for evaluation to assess the proximity of injury to the aorta and other anatomic structures. In cases where the extent of injury has been beyond 3mm from the aorta, it has been thought to be safe to reinitiate feeds.
- Repeat esophograms are indicated and should occur within 4 days of ingestion, or sooner if symptomatic.

Further Reading

1. National Capital Poison Center. Button battery ingestion guidelines. Available at https://www.poison.org/battery/guideline. Accessed March 12, 2020.
2. Sethia, R, Gibbs, H, Jacobs, IN, Reilly, JS, Rhoades, K, Jatana, KR. Current management of button battery injuries. *Laryngoscope Investig Otolaryngol.* 2021;6:549–563. https://doi.org/10.1002/lio2.535.
3. Jatana KR, Barron CL, Jacobs IN. Initial clinical application of tissue pH neutralization after esophageal button battery removal in children. *Laryngoscope.* 2019;129:1772–1776. https://doi.org/10.1002/lary.27904.
4. National Capital Poison Center. Button battery ingestion statistics. Available at https://www.poison.org/battery/stats. Accessed November 1, 2020.
5. Gao Y, Wang J, Ma J, Gao Y, Zhang T, Lei P, Xiong X. Management of button batteries in the upper gastrointestinal tract of children: Aacase-series study. *Medicine (Baltimore).* 2020 Oct 16;99(42):e22681. doi: 10.1097/MD.0000000000022681. PMID: 33080713; PMCID: PMC7571923.
6. The American Academy of Pediatrics, Button Battery Task Force. Available at https://www.aap.org/en-us/advocacy-and-policy/aap-health-initiatives/Pages/Button-Battery.aspx. Accessed October 17, 2020.
7. Sharpe SJ, Rochette LM, Smith GA. Pediatric battery-related emergency department visits in the United States, 1990–2009. *Pediatrics.* 2012;129:1111–1117.
8. Litovitz T, Whitaker N, Clark L, et al. Emerging battery-ingestion hazard: clinical implications. *Pediatrics.* 2010;125:1168–1177.
9. Leinwand K, Brumbaugh DE, Kramer RE. Button battery ingestion in children: a paradigm for management of severe pediatric foreign body ingestions. *Gastrointest Endosc Clin N Am.* 2016;26(1):99–118. doi:10.1016/j.giec.2015.08.003.
10. Litovitz T, Whitaker N, Clark L. Preventing battery ingestions: an analysis of 8648 cases. *Pediatrics.* 2010;125:1178–1183. https://doi.org/10.1542/peds.2009-3038.
11. Gibbs H, Rhoades K, Jatana KR, Clinical guidelines and advocacy for the reduction of pediatric button battery injuries. *Clin Pediatr Emerg Med.* 2020;21(2):100775, ISSN 1522–8401. https://doi.org/10.1016/j.cpem.2020.100775.

12. Tanaka J, Yamashita M, Kajigaya H. Esophageal electrochemical burns due to button type lithium batteries in dogs. *Vet Hum Toxicol*. 1998;40(4):193–196.

13. Jatana KR, Litovitz T, Reilly JS, et al. Pediatric button battery injuries: 2013 task force update. *Int J Pediatr Otorhinolaryngol*. 2013;77 (9):1392–1399.

14. National Capital Poison Center. Fatal button battery ingestions. Available at https://www.poison.org/battery/fatalcases. Accessed March 12, 2021.

15. Varga Á, Kovács T, Saxena AK. Analysis of complications after button battery ingestion in children. *Pediatr Emerg Care*. 2018 Jun;34(6):443–446. doi: 10.1097/ PEC.0000000000001413. PMID: 29369262.

16. Thabet MH, Basha WM, Askar S. Button battery foreign bodies in children: hazards, management, and recommendations. *Biomed Res Int*. 2013;2013:846091.

17. Kramer RE, Lerner DG, Lin T, et al. Management of ingested foreign bodies in children: a clinical report of the NASPGHAN Endoscopy Committee. *J Pediatr Gastroenterol Nutr*. 2015;60:562–574.

9 To Wheeze or Not to Wheeze

Linda Vachon and Emily Rose

Case Study

Parents bring in a previously healthy 18-month-old female with increased work of breathing. Symptoms began 5 days ago with a runny nose and mild cough, which progressed to increased work of breathing after 2 days. In the Emergency Department (ED), the child is slightly tachypneic, has mild retractions, but is maintaining her oxygenation at 97% and is able to tolerate liquids. Her urinary output is maintained, but parents note that her diapers are less full than usual. She had a mild fever initially which resolved after 3 days. However, this morning she developed a fever of 104°F, and parents noted that she had some grunting on the physical exam. Parents were concerned because the patient's twin sister was ill with the same symptoms (1–2 days earlier than the patient) and she has completely recovered and is without fever or significant respiratory symptoms. On a clinical exam, the patient has rhonchi throughout all lung fields.

What do you do now?

DIAGNOSIS

A runny nose and cough in a toddler-aged child is most commonly of viral etiology. Upper respiratory tract infections that progress to include the lower respiratory tract, especially in association with increased work of breathing in a toddler-aged child, are consistent with the clinical presentation of bronchiolitis. Due to the onset of a new fever in addition to the development of grunting, a chest x-ray is obtained to evaluate for development of an additional bacterial pneumonia complicating a viral bronchiolitis presentation. A urinalysis is also obtained for a secondary episode of fever during the illness in a female <24 months of age who is relatively at increased risk for a urinary tract infection (compared to a lower risk male >1 year of age).

Bronchiolitis is a seasonal clinical syndrome that commonly occurs in young children <2 years old. Approximately one-third of children have bronchiolitis in the first year of life, and 90% by 2 years of age. Many viruses can cause this clinical pattern, and not infrequently, more than one viral infection can occur concomitantly. Up to one-third of patients hospitalized with bronchiolitis have co-infection with more than one virus, and these patients may have a more severe or stuttering clinical course.

The classic clinical presentation of bronchiolitis is an infant or toddler with respiratory symptoms of varying severity. The morbidity of symptoms varies with the age of the patient, preexisting conditions/comorbidities, as well as disease course and patient's immune response. The viral infection induces respiratory epithelial necrosis and mucosal edema. This inflammation causes obstruction and increased work of breathing in the relatively small airways of infants and toddlers. This airway debris may even completely obstruct bronchioles and cause lobar collapse. In severe cases, this viral pneumonia may cause lung necrosis and permanent scarring.

Classically, patients experience 1–2 days of runny nose (upper respiratory tract involvement) and begin to develop lower respiratory tract symptoms on days 2–3 of illness. Peak severity of symptoms occurs during days 3–5 of illness. Tachypnea, retractions, nasal flaring, and increased work of breathing are common as the lower respiratory tract becomes involved. Diffuse wheezing or rales are commonly present on auscultation. Many infants have decreased oral intake secondary to nasal obstruction and difficulty breathing. Fever is often present, and a persistent cough (on average of 2 weeks) frequently occurs.

Chest radiographs are seldom necessary in children with classic signs and symptoms of bronchiolitis (see Box 9.1). A negative radiograph can also support withholding antibiotics. In general, a single supine anteroposterior (AP) view of the chest is sufficient. A lateral view can be helpful to clarify an abnormality seen on the AP view or to confirm hyperinflation. When evaluating the pediatric chest x-ray, it is important to review it systematically and to be cognizant of the differences based on age.

So a chest radiograph is obtained. How do you read a chest radiograph?

The approach to reading the chest x-ray of an infant is similar to that of an adult. An initial rapid assessment of the radiograph as a whole is helpful to determine which areas require additional scrutiny. This overview is followed by a systematic approach of first identifying any indwelling lines and tubes, followed by the soft tissues/bones, lungs/trachea, and bronchi and heart/mediastinum. Finally, the clinical information on the request is reviewed. This information is extremely important in creating a differential diagnosis and may necessitate another review of the radiograph.

There are several normal findings in the infant chest which are not seen in the adult. The most obvious finding is the thymus, which is largest in the first year of life. It is typically in the anterior mediastinum, blends imperceptibly with the cardiac silhouette, and causes no mass effect on the mediastinum (Figures 9.1a and 9.1b). Tracheal buckling, usually to the right, is another common finding on expiratory radiographs in infants and young children (Figure 9.2). If the trachea buckles to the left, a right-sided aortic arch or mass should be suspected. Lastly, the heart often appears enlarged in

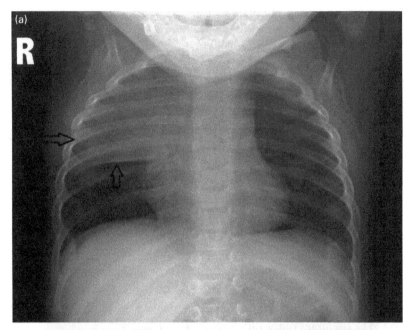

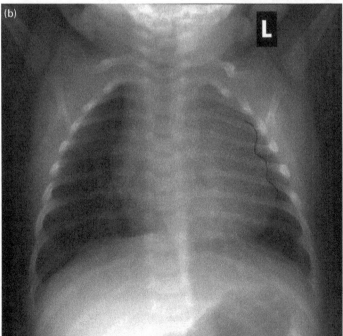

FIGURES 9.1a AND 9.1b. Features of the normal thymus. (a) Arrows point to the thymic "sail sign" which is often seen on the right. Note that the thymus has the same density as the heart. (b) The thymic "wave sign" is outlined and is due to compression of the thymus by the anterior ribs.

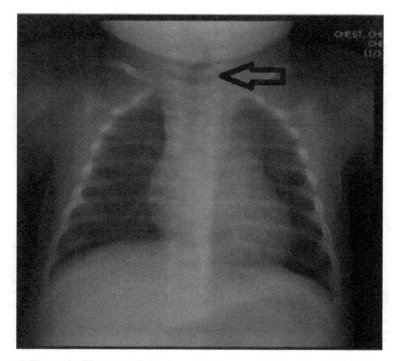

FIGURE 9.2. Tracheal buckling (arrow).

infants, especially on expiratory x-rays (Figures 9.3a and 9.3b). The cardio-thoracic ratio can be .55 in infants, compared to .50 in adults.

In viral bronchiolitis, the radiographic appearance is varied and is the result of inflammation affecting mainly the bronchial mucosa. The classic findings are usually diffuse and are typically described as hyperinfla-tion, peribronchial cuffing, and/or segmental or subsegmental atelectasis (Figure 9.4).

Hyperinflation in a child less than 3 years of age is noted if lung expan-sion is greater than the 9th posterior rib. A rapid way of assessing hyper-inflation is visualizing the heart border completely above the diaphragm. Flattening of the diaphragms is another clue to hyperinflation and can best be seen on the lateral view.

Peribronchial cuffing is noted when the wall of a peripheral bronchus, seen end on, is thickened and resembles a donut. The normal bronchial wall is the thickness of an eggshell.

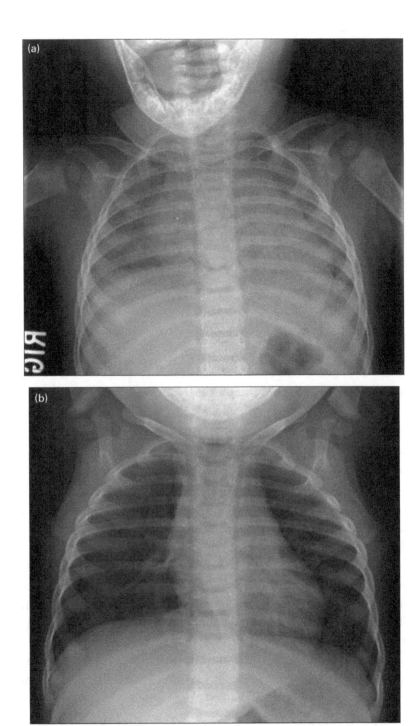

FIGURES 9.3a AND 9.3b. Infant suspected of having cardiomegaly based on initial x-ray.
(a) Initial expiratory chest x-ray. (b) Same patient with adequate inspiration.

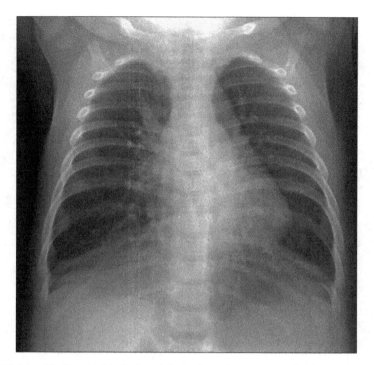

FIGURE 9.4. Viral bronchiolitis. The frontal chest radiograph shows hyperinflation to the level of the 10th posterior rib. There is no heart shadow below the diaphragm. Thick, linear opacities are seen in the right upper lobe medially and represent subsegmental atelectasis.

Segmental atelectasis and subsegmental atelectasis appear as central opacities with sharp borders, are usually multifocal, and change configuration rapidly on subsequent x-rays. Atelectasis is commonly mistaken for focal bacterial pneumonia, but although the findings often overlap, a singular, ill-defined peripheral opacity is more likely to be bacterial, especially if associated with a pleural effusion (Figure 9.5). Pleural effusions are uncommon in viral infections. In the neonatal period, bacterial infections are more common than viral and tend to be diffuse, mimicking a viral pattern.

The radiographic findings detailed above can aid in distinguishing viral from bacterial infections, but cannot alone reliably distinguish between them as viral pneumonias can appear as focal opacities and bacterial pneumonias can be diffuse and interstitial in the 2-month–2-year age group. However, acute bacterial superinfection of bronchiolitis is rare.

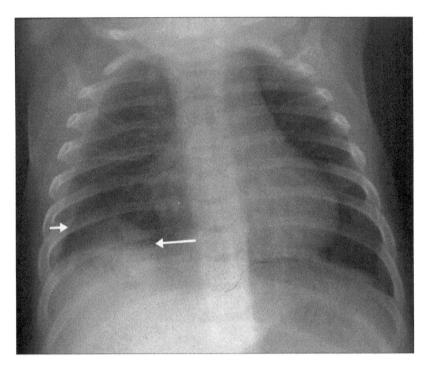

FIGURE 9.5. Pneumonia due to *S. aureus*. Frontal chest x-ray demonstrates focal, peripheral opacity in the right lower lobe (long arrow) with adjacent pleural effusion (small arrow).

Most children with bacterial pneumonia appear clinically ill and have moderate-significant fever. Onset of symptoms are fairly abrupt. Sepsis is more common with typical bacterial pneumonia than other etiologies of respiratory symptoms. Grunting is associated with significant airway disease and is often a sign of impending respiratory failure. Focal crackles, decreased breath sounds, dullness to percussion, and/or abnormal transmission of sounds are found on clinical examination. Wheezing is most typical in asthma and bronchiolitis, but may occur in viral and atypical bacterial pneumonia.

The epidemiology of pediatric pneumonia is impacted by age, vaccination status, and local immunization status of the surrounding community (herd immunity protection for those unvaccinated or too young to be vaccinated). Overall, 60%–90% of pediatric pneumonia is of viral etiology. Higher-risk age groups include the neonate, the immunocompromised, and those with significant comorbidities. Viruses are the most common cause of pneumonia in older infants, toddlers, and young children. Lobar pneumonia/"typical pneumonia" is most commonly caused by *Streptococcus pneumoniae* in all ages. The incidence has decreased with better vaccination coverage against *S. pneumoniae* strains. Atypical bacterial pneumonia infections due to mycoplasma are more common in children >5 years, though the relative prevalence has increased with improved vaccination coverage against *S. pneumoniae.* The true prevalence of various etiologies of community acquired pneumonia in children is unknown, and several recent studies have shown that the incidence of bacterial pneumonia in children is likely lower than previously thought.

Because bacterial superinfection of bronchiolitis is rare, the American Academy of Pediatrics recommends *against* the routine use of antibiotics in most patients. There are no medical therapies that have been proven to significantly impact the clinical course of patients with viral bronchiolitis. The cornerstone of management is suctioning and respiratory support as needed. Bronchiolitis is a significant cause of morbidity and mortality in children, so disposition should be carefully considered in those with risk factors for decompensation and complications. Risk factors include neonatal age, a history of prematurity, and those with comorbidities (including those with increased physiologic demand or decreased respiratory effort such as pulmonary, cardiac, neurologic disease or those with immunocompromise). Hydration status should also be assessed and dehydration treated.

Admission indications include patients with apnea, significant respiratory distress not responsive to suctioning, oxygen saturation <90%, tachypnea >60–80 breaths per minute, inability to tolerate liquids, or significant underlying cardiopulmonary or neurologic disease. A low threshold for admission should be maintained in the neonate, premature infant, and those with comorbidities or unstable social situations. Length of symptoms may help anticipate the disease course. A patient on day 1–2 of illness is likely to worsen and increase in clinical severity, whereas a patient on day 4–5 of illness is less likely to progress. Close follow-up is recommended for those with significant symptoms, particularly if seen early in their disease course, prior to peak severity.

Patients who are well-appearing, well-hydrated/able to tolerate feeds, without apnea, and not in respiratory distress with an oxygen saturation of >90% can be discharged home. Caregivers should monitor for signs of apnea, respiratory distress, and dehydration.

CASE CONCLUSION

In this patient's case, her x-ray was not significant for bacterial superinfection. Her urine did not show signs of infection. Her clinical appearance and respiratory status improved after suctioning and oral hydration during her ED course. Parents were given return precautions and she was discharged home with an appointment with her pediatrician the following morning. The clinical diagnosis was presumed to be a second viral infection with a bronchiolitis pattern.

KEY POINTS

- Bronchiolitis is a viral-induced clinical syndrome that occurs seasonally in children <2 years of age.
- The diagnosis of bronchiolitis is clinical. No viral testing or imaging is required.
- Risk factors for complications include <1 month of age, prematurity, comorbidities.
- Treatment is suctioning, respiratory support, and oxygen if needed.
- Admission should be considered for apneic episodes, hypoxia, respiratory distress, or poor oral intake. A low threshold for admission should be maintained for the neonate and those with comorbidities
- Children who are well appearing, well hydrated/tolerating orals with oxygen saturation>90% can be discharged home with good parental instructions.
- Etiology of pneumonia in children varies by age.
- Most pneumonia in young children is viral in etiology.

- Always check the positions of indwelling lines and tubes first.
- A single, focal consolidation is most likely a bacterial pneumonia.
- Diffuse, interstitial pneumonias are often viral, but bacterial pneumonias can have a similar appearance, especially in very young children.
- Pleural effusions are rare in viral pneumonias.
- Radiographic findings are poor indicators of etiology of pneumonia and cannot be relied upon entirely for diagnosis.

Further Reading

1. Balk DS, Lee C, Schafer J, Welwarth J, Hardin J, Novack V, Yarza S, Hoffmann B. Lung ultrasound compared to chest X-ray for diagnosis of pediatric pneumonia: a meta-analysis. *Pediatr Pulmonol*. 2018 Aug;53(8):1130–1139. doi: 10.1002/ppul.24020. Epub 2018 Apr 26. PMID: 29696826.

2. Messinger AI, Kupfer O, Hurst A, Parker S. Management of pediatric community-acquired bacterial pneumonia. *Pediatr Rev*. 2017 Sep;38(9):394–409. doi: 10.1542/pir.2016-0183. PMID: 28864731.

3. Lynch T, Gouin S, Larson C, Patenaude Y. Does the lateral chest radiograph help pediatric emergency physicians diagnose pneumonia? A randomized clinical trial. *Acad Emerg Med*. 2004; 11(6):625–9.

4. Claes AS, Clapuyt P, Menten R, Michoux N, Dumitriu D. Performance of chest ultrasound in pediatric pneumonia. *Eur J Radiol*. 2017 Mar;88:82–87. doi: 10.1016/j.ejrad.2016.12.032. Epub 2016 Dec 29. PMID: 28189214.

5. Rose E. Pediatric respiratory emergencies. In: Rose E, ed. *Pediatric Emergencies: A Practical, Clinical Guide*. New York: Oxford University Press; 2021:137–154.

6. Søndergaard MJ, Friis MB, Hansen DS, Jørgensen IM. Clinical manifestations in infants and children with Mycoplasma pneumoniae infection. *PLoS One*. 2018 Apr 26;13(4):e0195288. doi: 10.1371/journal.pone.0195288. PMID: 29698412; PMCID: PMC5919654.

10 I Thought They Fixed Me?

Gina Pizzitola, William Mak, and Rachelle Goldfisher

Case Study

A 7-year-old male presents to the emergency department 1 week after an appendectomy. He underwent a laparoscopic appendectomy after being diagnosed with an uncomplicated appendicitis. Last night he developed diffuse abdominal pain. He has vomited three times since this morning, which is described as yellow and is nonbloody, nonbilious. His mother reports that he has not stooled since the surgery and has had a poor appetite, only drinking a few cups of juice each day. He had been taking oxycodone for about 36 hours after surgery but since then has only been taking acetaminophen a couple of times per day. On arrival at the Emergency Department (ED) he appears uncomfortable but nontoxic. He is afebrile with a heart rate of 110 beats per minute and a blood pressure of 122/83mmHg. His abdomen is mildly distended and feels firm. The patient is diffusely tender to palpation, with more severe pain over the right lower quadrant. The surgical site is intact with no excessive erythema or drainage from the incision. The rest of his exam is unremarkable.

What do you do now?

DISCUSSION

In a child with recent abdominal surgery, symptoms of pain, fever, vomiting, or concerns regarding the surgical site should prompt further investigation. For the child described in this case, the presence of a painful, distended abdomen with vomiting necessitates urgent imaging and management, along with surgical consultation.

Complications after abdominal surgery can be very serious and should be diagnosed and addressed quickly in the ED. Rapid evaluation and diagnosis are especially important, as several postoperative complications can have similar presentations. Common presentations of complications include generalized abdominal pain, decreased appetite or oral intake, vomiting, and constipation. Often, it is the development of vomiting that alerts the clinician to the seriousness of the situation beyond simple postoperative pain. Radiographs are an important component in working up a postoperative patient with vomiting. The following discussion will help guide you through what is at times a vague presentation to the end of diagnosing life-threatening conditions while pursuing as little radiation as is reasonable.

In general, complications after abdominal surgery in children are rare. Possible complications include infection of the incision or intra-abdominal surgical site (including development of an abscess), postoperative ileus, constipation, and small bowel obstruction (SBO).

Postoperative ileus is often the normal response to abdominal intervention. Constipation may result from decreased oral intake, decreased activity, and the use of narcotic drugs for pain control. To help differentiate between ileus and constipation, a plain film series, with supine and upright (or decubitus) films, may be obtained. An x-ray with air-fluid levels (Figure 10.1) is concerning for some form of obstruction, including an ileus. Basic constipation should not have any air-fluid levels, but rather should show a significant stool burden with no other concerning features (such as free air).

The presence of air-fluid levels necessitates further workup, as this is concerning but not specific. Early in the postoperative course, air-fluid levels may be the result of postoperative ileus, which will likely resolve with time. However, they may also indicate an obstruction. In the near-postoperative period this may be due to a large abscess, severe constipation,

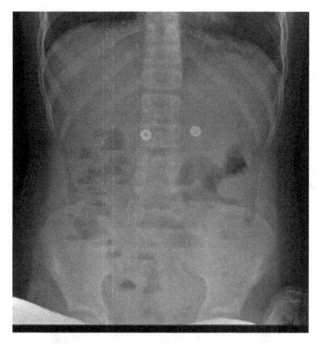

FIGURE 10.1. Upright frontal view of the abdomen demonstrates multiple air fluid levels. Air-fluid levels may be seen with an ileus or in small bowel obstruction.

or other surgical complication. Several weeks or more after surgery, this may be the result of adhesions. Regardless of etiology, the child with air-fluid levels warrants further evaluation with abdominal/pelvic computed tomography (CT) scan.

For patients presenting with fevers and focal pain near the surgical site but otherwise without signs of obstruction (stooling and tolerating oral intake without emesis), and in which the development of an abscess is highly suspected, one may consider initial imaging with ultrasound. The finding of a discrete hypoechoic collection near the surgical site would support this diagnosis and prompt discussion with surgery for definitive management.

Although rare, another possible complication of abdominal surgery is intestinal perforation. Plain films are also the first line. You may consider adding a lateral decubitus film for the postoperative vomiting child that has a distended taut belly. A positive film will reveal free air (black) beneath the diaphragm. While soon after surgery this may be left over from operative insufflation, it can also suggest a perforation. Residual gas from an operative insufflation is almost always reabsorbed within 5 days.[1] If there is sufficient concern for perforation, you should immediately consult surgery or transfer the child to a facility with surgical capabilities.

When obtaining a CT scan to evaluate for SBO, you may use oral contrast if the patient is able to tolerate it. One study showed that CT had good sensitivity and specificity for SBO, but not necessarily for determination of the cause of SBO.[2] It is important to note that a CT scan may not reliably differentiate between an ileus and SBO.[3] Nevertheless, a CT may help guide the consulting surgical team in continued management of the patient. CT imaging has the additional benefit of characterizing the underlying condition and may reveal the location of the obstruction or the presence of an abscess (Figures 10.2 and 10.3).[4]

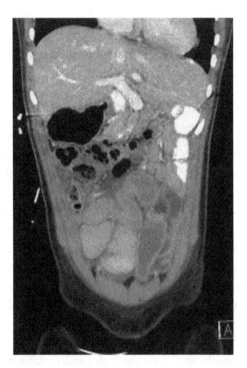

FIGURE 10.2. Coronal contrast enhanced CT image demonstrates multiple dilated bowel loops with diluted oral contrast.

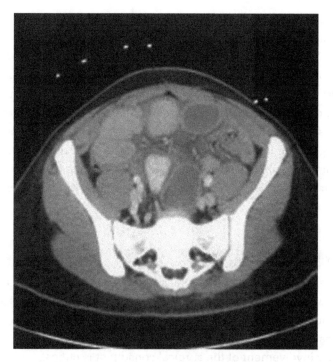

FIGURE 10.3. Axial CT image obtained following oral and IV contrast administration which demonstrates multiple dilated bowel loops in this case of postoperative small bowel obstruction (SBO).

In an effort to limit a child's lifetime exposure to radiation, it may be acceptable to pursue magnetic resonance imaging (MRI) of the abdomen and pelvis in lieu of a CT scan, but only if the modality is readily available.[4] If it has been determined, however, that a child requires advanced imaging to rule out emergent intervention, it is not appropriate to delay imaging to decrease radiation risk. In such a case, a CT scan should be obtained as soon as possible.

Case Conclusion

The patient's exam continued to be reassuring without guarding or rigidity. Radiographs were obtained on the patient in the scenario and showed a lack of air-fluid levels, absence of free air, and presence of significant stool on imaging. The patient's use of narcotics and lack of stooling are consistent with constipation for the patient in the scenario. This child will likely benefit from a bowel regimen and perhaps an enema.

It is important to consult surgery early in the patient's course. Most of these conditions will require close monitoring by the surgical team (as in the case of postoperative ileus) and sometimes surgical intervention (for example, to lyse adhesions). It may also be necessary to bring in other teams (such as interventional radiology to drain an abscess). In such cases, the imaging modalities you select may not solely help determine the etiology, but can help them with approach (for example, locating the abscess). Early consultations with supportive imaging can help these team members create their treatment plans.

KEY POINTS

- Complications after abdominal surgery in children are rare and include infection of the incision or intra-abdominal surgical site (including development of an abscess), postoperative ileus, constipation, and SBO.
- Early involvement of the surgical consultant is critical.

TIPS FROM THE RADIOLOGIST

- An abdominal plain film series is an important first step in determining the presence of SBO.
- Signs of SBO include air fluid levels and dilated loops of bowel.
- CT scan is highly reliable in differentiating complete SBO from ileus, but less reliable in differentiating ileus from partial SBO.
- When concerned about perforation, it is important to obtain a lateral decubitus or upright abdominal plain film.
- Ultrasound may be used as an initial tool to evaluate the child presenting with fevers and focal pain near the surgical site (without signs of obstruction) to look for an abscess.

References

1. Tallant C, et al. Spontaneous pneumoperitoneum in pediatric patients: a case series. *Int J Surg Case Rep.* 2016;22:55–58. doi:10.1016/j.ijscr.2016.03.017.

2. Jabra AA, et al. CT of small-bowel obstruction in children. *Am J Roentgenol*. 2001;177(2):431–436. https://www.ajronline.org/doi/full/10.2214/ajr.177.2.1770431.
3. Frager DH, et al. Distinction between postoperative ileus and mechanical small-bowel obstruction: value of CT compared with clinical and other radiographic findings. *Am J Roentgenol*. 1995;164:891–894. https://www.ajronline.org/doi/pdf/10.2214/ajr.164.4.7726042.
4. American College of Radiology. ACR Appropriateness Criteria® suspected small-bowel obstruction. acsearch.acr.org. https://acsearch.acr.org/docs/69476/Narrative/. Revised 2019.

Weebly, Wobbly

Meika Eby, Nkeiruka Orajiaka, and Lauren May

Case Study

A 13-year-old male with no past medical history presents to the Emergency Department (ED) for left leg pain and limping. The pain began a few days ago in his left knee and thigh, waxes and wanes but does not radiate. The pain has progressed and is now associated with a limp. He is active in football and denies any recent or past trauma. He presents for evaluation due to worsening symptoms after practice today. He denies fever, systemic symptoms, and recent illness. On exam, he is 62 inches tall and weighs 150 pounds (BMI 97th percentile) with normal vitals. Lower extremity exam is remarkable for pain with range of motion at the left hip, worse with internal rotation, as well as slight external rotation when flexing the hip. His knee exam is normal. There is no point tenderness, swelling, or discoloration and he is neurovascularly intact. His gait is slightly antalgic, but the remainder of the exam is otherwise normal.

What do you do now?

DISCUSSION

In the pediatric patient with hip pain, several differential diagnoses should be entertained including slipped capital femoral epiphysis (SCFE, a Salter-Harris I fracture of the sub-capital femoral physis), pelvic apophyseal avulsion fracture, traumatic pelvic or proximal femoral fracture, juvenile idiopathic arthritis, septic arthritis, toxic synovitis, muscular strain/spasm, malignancy, and Legg-Calve-Perthes (LCP) disease. History and physical exam can be paramount in narrowing this differential prior to further workup, which may include radiographic or laboratory studies. In this case, the patient is an overweight adolescent with subacute to chronic pain that is worsening and occurs with athletic participation. Therefore, the top two differential diagnoses to include would be SCFE and pelvic apophyseal avulsion fracture. A pelvic radiograph (also referred to as bilateral hip radiograph) would be appropriate for the next step in workup.

In all pediatric patients with unilateral or bilateral hip pain, initial pelvic radiographs should include two views: an anteroposterior (AP) view and a lateral view (frog-leg), with each image including the entire pelvis and both proximal femurs. Views of both hips are required because both SCFE and pelvic apophyseal avulsion fractures can be bilateral. Additionally, viewing the contralateral pelvis and hip can be valuable in assessing for subtle asymmetric findings, such as a pre-slip SCFE or a nondisplaced pelvic apophyseal avulsion fracture that might otherwise be overlooked.

SLIPPED CAPITAL FEMORAL EPIPHYSIS (SCFE)

SCFE occurs when the femoral epiphysis is displaced relative to the femoral neck through the physis (growth plate). It is the most common hip disorder among adolescents, typically ages 10–14 years old with the average age of onset around 12 years old (slightly older in males and younger in females). There is a slight male predominance (approximately 1.5:1) and higher prevalence in Blacks, Hispanics, Polynesians, and Native Americans. Predisposing factors have been attributed to changes in the physis such as increased stress and weakening, which correlate with known risk factors for SCFE such as obesity, metabolic abnormalities (e.g., hypothyroidism), and puberty.

Awareness of varying presentations is key as delayed diagnosis can lead to poorer long-term outcomes such as extensive cartilage damage, secondary osteoarthritis, and avascular necrosis. One study showed that up to 75% of cases had been seen previously at their primary care facility for relevant symptoms and others have noted weeks to months in delay of diagnosis. Patients typically present with hip, thigh, or knee pain, limping, difficulty or inability to bear weight, or a combination of symptoms. The pain can be acute, subacute, or chronic, as well as unilateral or bilateral. The pain also may be constant or only with walking. Bilateral SCFE occurs in 18%–63% of cases, but only half of those may initially present with bilateral pain.

Appropriate physical exam is necessary for diagnosis. The patient should be supine when examining the hip, and the hip should *always* be examined in patients complaining of knee pain. The most common finding is limited internal rotation of the affected hip. Other typical exam findings include decreased passive range of motion of the hip, especially flexion, and limping in stable SCFE (unstable SCFE patients are not able to bear weight). A positive Drehmann sign is suggestive of SCFE and is described as obligatory external rotation and abduction when passively flexing the affected hip.

In the majority of patients, only pelvic radiographs are required. You obtain radiographs of the pelvis in your patient. In this patient there are typical findings of an SCFE (Figures 11.1a and 11.1b). On the AP view there is abnormal asymmetric widening of the left sub-capital femoral physis. On the AP view of a patient without SCFE, a line drawn along the lateral femoral

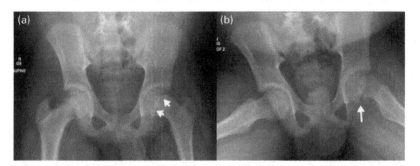

FIGURES 11.1a AND 11.1b. AP (a) and frog-leg (b) views of the pelvis demonstrate a slipped capital femoral epiphysis in the left hip. There is widening of the physis (small arrows in a) and slippage of the epiphysis medially and posteriorly with respect to the metaphysis (arrow in b).

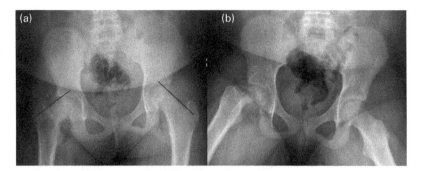

FIGURES 11.2a AND 11.2b. SCFE in another patient. AP (a) and frog-leg (b) views of the pelvis. The Klein line (black line in a) drawn parallel to the lateral/upper border of the femoral neck fails to intersect the femoral epiphysis on the right side compared to the left side. The SCFE is better seen on the frog leg view on the right side.

neck (known as a Klein line) should intersect the outer femoral head. In a patient with SCFE, the Klein line will cross lateral to the slipped femoral capital femoral epiphysis (Figures 11.2a and 11.2b). SCFE is often easier to identify on the frog-leg view because the femoral head epiphysis typically displaces posteriorly and medially relative to the femoral metaphysis (Figures 11.1a and 11.b and Figures 11.2a and 11.2.b). In chronic SCFE, the metaphysis may be irregular, sclerotic, scalloped, or may show posterior beaking. Rarely, the epiphysis can displace laterally and superiorly, known as a valgus SCFE. In the case of a pre-slip there may be no significant displacement of the capital physis, and the only indication may be widening of the physis with irregularity and osseous remodeling of the metaphysis.

Magnetic resonance imaging (MRI) is more sensitive, especially in the setting of pre-slip SCFE, but is rarely required during the initial assessment. MRI may show widening of the physis, marrow edema, synovitis, and an effusion. MRI may be more helpful to assess long-term outcome after treatment, especially if there is concern for femoro-acetabular impingement, labral tear, articular cartilage damage, or avascular necrosis.

A diagnosis of SCFE, especially if unstable, warrants an immediate orthopedic consult as the treatment is surgical stabilization. The patient should be made non-weight-bearing until surgical intervention. Standard treatment consists of screw fixation. If the SCFE is stable or mildly displaced, fixation can be performed percutaneously without femoral head manipulation. If there is moderate to severe displacement and/or instability, open capital realignment and screw fixation may be warranted. However, manual reduction of the femoral capital epiphysis is associated with a higher risk of avascular necrosis. Prophylactic contralateral fixation is controversial but may be considered, especially for patients who have a predisposition for contralateral SCFE.

LEGG-CALVE-PERTHES (LCP)

A differential diagnosis for SCFE is Legg-Calve-Perthes (LCP). This is a developmental condition that causes necrosis of the femoral head. It is one of the most common causes of permanent femoral head deformity in childhood and affects children between 3–12 years of age, with a peak at 5–7 years of age. LCP is 3 to 4 times more likely to affect boys than girls. The incidence also varies depending on socioeconomic class, with LCP being more common in less densely populated areas and lower socioeconomic classes.

The etiology of LCP has been widely studied but is still not clearly understood. Several hypotheses have proposed that it is multifactorial, involving genetic, mechanical, and systemic components. The best-supported theory purports that genetic factors confer susceptibility to the disruption of the blood supply to the capital femoral epiphysis and that environmental factors, such as repeated subclinical trauma resulting from hyperactivity or mechanical overload, trigger the disease.

Early recognition and diagnosis of LCP is important, as patients in whom the disease presents before the age of 5–7 years have been found to have a substantially better outcome than those presenting after age 8–9 years. Children with LCP present with mild hip pain which often refers to the antero-medial thigh or knee, and a Trendelenburg gait. On examination, patients may have limited internal rotation and abduction of the hip. Radiographs in the earliest stage may be negative, but over time sclerosis, subchondral fracture, fragmentation, and eventually healing of the femoral head will be seen depending on the stage of disease (Figures 11.3a and 11.3b).

When diagnosed in the ED, children should be made non-weight-bearing with use of crutches and referred to an experienced pediatric orthopedic specialist for management. Management options vary, but generally focus on containing the femoral head within the acetabulum with either

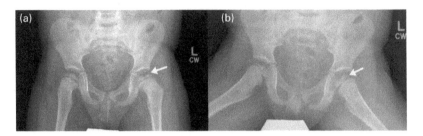

FIGURES 11.3a AND 11.3b. AP (a) and frog-leg (b) views of the pelvis in a patient with left sided Legg-Calve-Perthes disease. The left femoral epiphysis is smaller, more sclerotic, and fragmented (arrow).

non-operative and/or operative interventions. The prognosis of the hip joint affected by LCP depends on the age of the patient at the time of onset, the stage of the disease, the extent of epiphyseal involvement, and the lateral extrusion of the femoral head.

Tips for Reading Pelvic Films

1. Image the entire pelvis with AP and frog-leg views to identify subtle asymmetric findings, such as a SCFE pre-slip or a nondisplaced avulsion fracture.
2. Trace cortical margins for disruption, buckling, or irregularities that will signify fractures, lesions, avascular necrosis, or erosions.
3. Assess all joints, including the sacroiliac joints, pubic symphysis, and hips.
4. Be familiar with basic lines that help assess alignment, such as Klein line and Shenton's arc.
5. Assess common sites of pelvic avulsion injuries, including the anterior superior iliac spine, anterior inferior iliac spine, and ischial tuberosity, as well as other less common sites of pelvic avulsion fractures.
6. When ordering pelvic radiographs, a specific history detailing a focal complaint is extremely helpful to the radiologist, rather than a generalized order history such as "hip pain." There are many structures evaluated on a pelvic radiograph, and a detailed history can improve the sensitivity and specificity of the radiology report.

Case Conclusion

Our patient presented with common symptoms concerning for SCFE: acute to subacute onset, referred pain from the knee, limping, decreased hip range of motion, and a positive Drehmann's sign. He had multiple risk factors, including being an adolescent, obese, and male. Confounding factors such as sports involvement may lead to a misdiagnosis of muscular strain/sprain even in the absence of a known traumatic injury. Therefore, clinical suspicion based on appropriate history, physical exam, and imaging was key in preventing morbidity and mortality. The patient was kept non-weight-bearing and was admitted to the hospital to orthopedics for operative intervention. He was discharged 2 days later and underwent physical therapy for a full recovery.

KEY POINTS

- SCFE typically presents in 10–14-year-old patients and can present with acute, subacute, or chronic pain, and can be unilateral or bilateral.
- Hip examination is important as many patients with SCFE or LCP present with referred pain in the knee or thigh.
- LCP is one of the most common causes of permanent femoral head damage in children.

TIPS FROM THE RADIOLOGIST

- Always include bilateral hip/entire pelvis on imaging. SCFE can present bilaterally or can be subtle in the case of a pre-slip making contralateral hip evaluation helpful.
- Frog-leg views demonstrate SCFE better than AP views.
- Diagnosis of LCP in early stages requires a high index of suspicion as initial radiographs may be normal. MRI may be needed in some cases.

Further Reading

1. Merrow AC, Linscott LL, O'Hara SM. Slipped capital femoral epiphysis. In: Merrow AC, Linscott LL, O'Hara. *Diagnostic Imaging Pediatrics*. 3rd ed. Elsevier; 2017:942–945.

2. Takao M, Hashimoto J, Sakai T, et al. Metaphyseal bone collapse mimicking slipped capital femoral epiphysis in severe renal osteodystrophy. *J Clin Endocrinol Metab.* 2012;97(11):3851–3856.

3. Karkenny AJ, Tauberg BM, Otsuka NY. Pediatric hip disorders: slipped capital femoral epiphysis and Legg-Calvé-Perthes disease. *Pediatr Rev.* 2018;39(9):454–463. doi: 10.1542/pir.2017-0197.

4. Uvodich M, Schwend R, Stevanovic O, Wurster W, Leamon J, Hermanson A. Patterns of pain in adolescents with slipped capital femoral epiphysis. *J Pediatr.* 2019;206:184–189.e1. doi: 10.1016/j.jpeds.2018.10.050.

5. Lehmann CL, Arons RR, Loder RT, Vitale MG. The epidemiology of slipped capital femoral epiphysis: an update. *J Pediatr Orthop.* 2006;26(3):286–290. doi: 10.1097/01.bpo.0000217718.10728.70

6. Loder RT, Skopelja EN. The epidemiology and demographics of slipped capital femoral epiphysis. *ISRN Orthop.* 2011 Sep 21;2011:486512. doi: 10.5402/2011/486512.

7. Millis MB. SCFE: clinical aspects, diagnosis, and classification. *J Child Orthop.* 2017;11(2):93–98. doi: 10.1302/1863-2548-11-170025.

8. Novais EN, Millis MB. Slipped capital femoral epiphysis: prevalence, pathogenesis, and natural history. *Clin Orthop Relat Res.* 2012;470(12):3432–3438. doi: 10.1007/s11999-012-2452-y.

9. Otani T, Kawaguchi Y, Marumo K. Diagnosis and treatment of slipped capital femoral epiphysis: recent trends to note. *J Orthop Sci.* 2018;23(2):220–228. doi: 10.1016/j.jos.2017.12.009.

10. Guerado E, Caso E. The physiopathology of avascular necrosis of the femoral head: an update. *Injury.* 2016;47 Suppl 6:S16–S26. doi: 10.1016/S0020-1383(16)30835-X.

11. Pavone V, Chisari E, Vescio A, Lizzio C, Sessa G, Testa G. Aetiology of Legg-Calvé-Perthes disease: a systematic review. *World J Orthop.* 2019 Mar 18;10(3):145–165. doi:10.5312/wjo.v10.i3.145

12. Ibrahim T, Little DG. The pathogenesis and treatment of Legg-Calvé-Perthes disease. *JBJS Rev.* 2016;4(7):e4. doi: 10.2106/JBJS.RVW.15.00063.

12 Extreme Extremity

Waroot S. Nimjareansuk and Jane S. Kim

Case Study

An 11-year-old female presents to the Emergency Department (ED) after a running accident. Earlier, she was running with her friends when she tripped, twisted her ankle, and fell on her outstretched hand. She reports immediate pain and swelling in both the wrist and ankle. On physical examination, there is swelling and tenderness to palpation at the level of the distal radius, with difficulty in pronation/supination maneuvers and soft tissue swelling and tenderness to palpation along the distal tibia. No signs of neurovascular injury are present. The patient is unable to bear weight on the ankle and has swelling and tenderness. Neurovascular exam is intact. An x-ray of the wrist and ankle are ordered (Figures 12.1 and 12.2).

What do you do now?

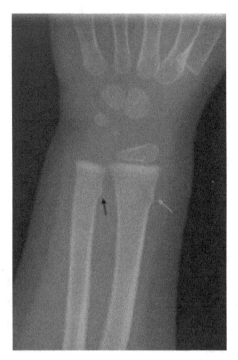

FIGURE 12.1. Radiograph of the wrist shows a torus fracture at the metaphysis on the medial aspect of the distal radius (white arrow), and an additional torus fracture at the metaphysis on the medial aspect of the distal ulna (black arrow).

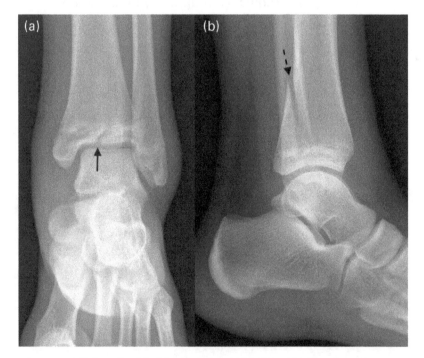

FIGURE 12.2. Radiographs of the left ankle in frontal (a) and lateral (b) views show a fracture lucency through the distal tibial epiphysis (black arrow) and a fracture lucency through the posterior distal tibial metaphysis (dotted black arrow) in a classic Triplane configuration.

DISCUSSION

Pediatric extremity fractures are common musculoskeletal injuries presenting to the ED. Increased bone elasticity, comparably stronger ligaments, and the presence of the physeal growth plates lead to unique fracture patterns in children. The differential diagnosis in this case for the wrist injury includes torus fractures, greenstick fractures, Salter Harris fractures, and scaphoid fractures. The differential diagnosis in this case for the ankle injury includes Triplane fracture, Juvenile Tillaux fracture, posterior malleolar fracture, avulsion fractures, and ligamentous injury. In this chapter, we discuss the most common extremity fractures unique to the pediatric population.

Torus (Buckle) Fracture

The torus fracture is a common fracture in the pediatric population, almost always occurring in the long bones. The distal radius is the most frequent site of torus fractures, usually occurring at the metaphysis. The metaphyseal region is the most at risk because the cortex of the distal radius is relatively thin in this region. These injuries often occur between the ages of 7 and 12 years but can occur throughout all pediatric ages.

The most common mechanism for a torus fracture is an axial force, usually caused by a fall on an outstretched hand (FOOSH). Due to the inherent increased bone elasticity in the pediatric population, there is a greater propensity for the bone to bow or bend before breaking. The cortex will bulge out or in on the compression side and is usually intact on the tension side.

Anteroposterior (AP) and lateral views of the wrist are required to determine the level of cortical breach and the amount of displacement. The cortex of the diaphysis and metaphysis of long bones should be smooth. A buckle fracture will manifest on radiographs as either an outward cortical bump or angulation/indentation, usually accompanied by overlying soft tissue swelling. Figure 12.1 shows a torus fracture in our patient. It is imperative to look at all views provided, as often a buckle fracture may be subtle and manifest on a single view only. Moreover, the adjacent long bone should be carefully scrutinized for an additional fracture, often a buckle, greenstick, or even a plastic bowing deformity. Contralateral limb x-rays may be helpful to compare the normal extremity to the injured extremity to determine the presence of a plastic bowing fracture.

Torus fractures can be treated with a removable volar splint or cast. Several studies have shown that splinting resulted in a quicker return to function with no adverse effects compared to casting. These fractures heal well as they are inherently stable and often require only 2–4 weeks of immobilization, with healing guided by tenderness to the site. The fracture is usually examined at 2–3 weeks after injury. If there is no tenderness, then the patient can discontinue the splint and begin range of motion of the wrist.

Overall, there is very little risk of displacement given inherent stability of the torus fracture. In addition, complications are very rare.

Greenstick Fracture

Greenstick fractures are common and usually occur in children under 10 years of age, but also may occur in any age group. These fractures most commonly occur in the long bones, with most seen in the radius or ulna. In a greenstick fracture, the cortex and periosteum are only disrupted on a single side of the bone, but remain intact on the other side. These injuries can be located along any portion of the metaphysis or diaphysis, but do not involve the physis (Salter-Harris fractures).

The physical examination usually reveals tenderness and swelling at the fracture site. It is important to assess the joint above and below the fracture site, along with a thorough neurovascular examination.

The mechanism of injury is usually a FOOSH or direct trauma, such as being hit by a hockey stick. The fall on an extended wrist can cause tension on the volar intercarpal and radiocarpal ligaments. In the pediatric population, the ligaments are usually stronger than bone, thus causing disruption of the bone while the ligaments remain intact.

AP and lateral views of the wrist are needed to determine the level of cortical disruption and the amount of displacement. Radiographs will reveal a fracture line on the tension side, not extending to the opposite cortex, which is intact. This is analogous to attempting to snap an immature "green" tree branch, where one side remains intact. In addition, there may be associated angulation present. In the distal radius, this translates into apex volar angulation and compression of the dorsal cortex. Again, it is imperative to scrutinize the adjacent long bone for additional fractures.

Treatment depends upon the degree of angulation and the location of the fracture. If there is significant angulation, then the fracture must be reduced and immobilized. For distal radius greenstick fractures, acceptable angulation should not exceed more than 20 degrees of dorsal angulation or 15 degrees of lateral angulation in boys under 9 years of age. The acceptable angulation for girls under 9 years of age is 5 degrees less than for boys at the same age. The acceptable angulation decreases by 5 degrees for every 2- to 3-year increase. Greenstick fractures can be immobilized in a sugar-tong splint with the elbow flexed to 90 degrees and the forearm and wrist in neutral position. All greenstick fractures require orthopedic referral given the risk of displacement or refracture. Typically, long bone greenstick fractures require casting for about 6 weeks, but the duration depends on the angulation and location of the fracture.

Although there is a risk of displacement, refracture, or complete fracture if not immobilized appropriately, the prognosis of greenstick fractures is still good as most of these fractures will heal without loss of function or significant deformity.

Salter-Harris Fracture

Salter-Harris fractures are common and account for 15%–30% of all childhood fractures. Salter-Harris fractures are fractures involving the physis or cartilaginous growth plate, located at the junction of the metaphysis and epiphysis. As a cartilaginous structure, the physis is a weak part of the bone, compared to the surrounding ligaments and capsular structures. Physeal injuries tend to occur in active children during the time of growth spurt, with a peak age of 11–12 years of age.

Salter-Harris fractures are classified into 5 subtypes, depending on the site of involvement (Figure 12.3). Type I involves only the physis; type II involves the physis and metaphysis; type III involves the physis and epiphysis; type IV involves the physis, metaphysis, and epiphysis; type V is a severe crush fracture involving the physis (Figure 12.3). A commonly used mnemonic for the classification system is SALTR: Slipped (type I), Above (type II), Lower (type III), Transverse/Through (type IV), and Ruined/Rammed (type V). Salter-Harris type II fracture is the most common (75%), followed by type III (10%), type IV (10%), type I (5%), and type V (very rare). Overall, Salter-Harris fractures occur more frequently in the upper extremities, with the distal radius the most common bone injured (28%), followed by the fingers (26%).

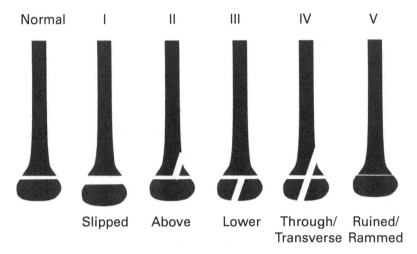

| Normal | I | II | III | IV | V |

Slipped   Above   Lower   Through/   Ruined/
                             Transverse Rammed

FIGURE 12.3. Salter-Harris classification diagram.

Courtesy of Andrew Phelps, MD.

Following a traumatic event, patients often present with pain, swelling, and point tenderness. Upper extremity injuries may result in immobility, and lower extremity injuries may result in inability to bear weight. Symptoms may mimic ligamentous injury.

Radiographs are the mainstay of diagnosis and may show metaphyseal and/or epiphyseal fracture lines extending to the physis. The physis, which is normally uniformly undulating, may be widened or interrupted. Ossification centers, including the medial malleolus and distal fibula, may be mistaken for fracture fragments. Obtaining radiographs of the contralateral side can be helpful for comparison purposes. It is important to be aware that Salter-Harris type I fractures may be radiographically occult.

In particular cases, computed tomography (CT) may be used to further define the fracture in terms of comminution, displacement, or articular involvement. Ultrasound may be useful in young infants with unossified cartilaginous epiphysis in determining displacement. Magnetic resonance imaging (MRI) is rarely employed but may be used to diagnose radiographically occult fractures, associated soft tissue injuries, or to evaluate for entrapment of periosteum after reduction.

Treatment depends on the fracture type, location, and degree of displacement, with Salter-Harris type I and II displaced fractures generally treated with closed reduction and casting. Salter-Harris type III and IV fractures involving the articular surface often require open reduction and internal fixation.

The overall complication rate is approximately 14%. Premature physeal closure with subsequent bony bridge formation may result in limb shortening and/or angulation. Intra-articular involvement may lead to joint incongruity and premature degenerative joint disease. Salter-Harris fractures of the lower extremity (distal femur and tibia) have a significant risk of growth disturbances (>50% for distal femur physeal injuries; 5%–50% for distal tibia physeal injuries). Therefore, it is imperative to obtain clinical and radiographic follow-up after the initial injury.

Triplane Fracture

Ankle injuries are the second most common site of injury in children 10–15 years of age, following hand and wrist injuries. Ankle fractures are twice as common in males, and represent 9%–18% of all physeal injuries. Triplane fractures are complex traumatic Salter-Harris type IV fractures involving the metaphysis, physis, and epiphysis of the distal tibia. These fractures typically occur in adolescents between 12 and 15 years of age, during the time period of tibial growth plate closure.

Closure of the tibial growth plate occurs in a predictable pattern, beginning in the central portion called "Kump's bump" in the medial edge of the talar hump. Progressive fusion first occurs in the posteromedial and then anterolateral direction. During this time of growth plate closure, the unfused portions of the physis are at risk for fracture, with lateral fractures more common than medial fractures. This same mechanism can result in a Juvenile Tillaux fracture, a Salter-Harris type III fracture of the distal tibial epiphysis caused by distraction of the anterior tibiofibular ligament.

Patients will often report a twisting injury while playing sports, resulting in pain and inability to bear weight. The most common mechanism of injury is external rotation with supination leading to the lateral triplane fracture type. The uncommon medial triplane fracture type may be caused by adduction. Swelling and tenderness to palpation are commonly appreciated on physical examination. Rarely, gross instability or angular deformity may be present.

There are several different triplane fracture configurations (2-part, 3-part, or 4-part), with or without intra-articular involvement. The classic triplane 3-plane fracture pattern (Figure 12.2) includes a coronal fracture plane through the tibial metaphysis (best seen on the lateral view), transverse fracture plane through the growth plate (which may be widened), and sagittal fracture plane through the epiphysis (best seen on the AP view). The ankle mortise view may be helpful in appreciating articular displacement. Triplane fractures may also be associated with fibular fractures in up to 50% of cases. A CT may be performed to further define the fracture planes, intra-articular involvement/step-off, and aid with presurgical planning.

Treatment depends on the fracture configuration, degree of displacement, and presence of intra-articular involvement. Most 2-part extra-articular fractures with less than 2mm displacement may be treated with non-operative management of closed reduction with internal rotation of the foot and long leg cast immobilization. Operative treatment with screw and/or K wire fixation may be indicated in 3-part fractures or if there is greater than 2mm displacement and/or articular step-off. Although physeal arrest may occur in 7%–21% of cases, this rarely leads to angular deformity. Prognosis is generally excellent, allowing for early identification and appropriate treatment.

The patient in our case underwent non-operative casting of the torus buckle fractures of the wrist (Figure 12.1). Due to the degree of displacement of the triplane ankle fracture (Figure 12.2) and mild intra-articular step-off, the patient underwent surgical reduction and screw fixation, with cast placement.

KEY POINTS

· The torus fracture almost exclusively occurs in pediatric long bones, with the wrist being the most common site.
· Torus fractures should be treated in a removable volar splint, and clinical healing should be guided by tenderness to the fracture site.

- Prompt immobilization and reduction beforehand, if needed, are of utmost importance as greenstick fractures can be unstable, leading to risk of refracture.
- There are 5 subtypes for Salter-Harris fractures, depending on site of involvement, with Salter-Harris type II fractures of the metaphysis and physis the most common type (75%).
- Intra-articular Salter-Harris type III and IV fractures will generally require surgical treatment.
- Triplane fractures occur in adolescents around the time of tibial growth plate closure.

TIPS FROM THE RADIOLOGIST

- In pediatric extremity radiography, developing ossification centers may be mistaken for fracture fragments. Obtaining radiographs of the contralateral side can often be helpful for comparison when in doubt.
- A CT scan may be helpful for triplane fractures to define the fracture planes and intra-articular involvement, and to aid with presurgical planning.

Further Reading

1. Asokan A, Kheir N. Pediatric torus buckle fracture. In: *StatPearls*. Treasure Island, FL: StatPearls; 2022. Available from: https://www.ncbi.nlm.nih.gov/books/NBK560 634/. August 16, 2020.
2. Eiff MP, Hatch R. *Fracture Management for Primary Care*. Philadelphia, PA: Elsevier Saunders; 2018.
3. Jiang N, Cao ZH, Ma YF, Lin Z, Yu B. Management of pediatric forearm torus fractures: a systematic review and meta-analysis. *Pediatr Emerg Care*. 2016;32(11):773–778. doi: 10.1097/PEC.0000000000000579.
4. Atanelov Z, Bentley TP. Greenstick fracture. In: *StatPearls*. Treasure Island, FL: StatPearls; 2022. August 26, 2020.
5. Noonan KJ, Price CT. Forearm and distal radius fractures in children. *J Am Acad Orthop Surg*. 1998;6(3):146–156. doi:10.5435/00124635-199805000-00002
6. Franklin CC, Robinson J, Noonan K, Flynn JM. Evidence-based medicine: management of pediatric forearm fractures. *J Pediatr Orthop*. 2012;32 Suppl 2:S131–S134. doi: 10.1097/BPO.0b013e318259543b.

7. Binkley A, Mehlman CT, Freeh E. Salter-Harris II ankle fractures in children: does fracture pattern matter? *J Orthop Trauma*. 2019;33(5):e190–e195.
8. Thomas RA, Hennrikus WL. Treatment and outcomes of distal tibia Salter Harris II fractures. *Injury*. 2020;51(3):636–641.
9. Jalkanen J, Sinikumpu JJ, Puhakka J, et al. Physeal Fractures of distal tibia: a systematic review and meta-analysis. *J Pediatr Orthop*. 2021. doi: 10.1097/BPO.0000000000001833. Epub ahead of print. PMID: 33843787.
10. Gaudiani MA, Knapik DM, Liu RW. Clinical outcomes of triplane fractures based on imaging modality utilization and management: a systematic review and meta-analysis. *J Pediatr Orthop*. 2020;40(10):e936–e941.
11. Solove M, Turcotte Benedict F. Ankle injuries in the Pediatric Emergency Department. *Pediatr Emerg Care*. 2020;36(5):248–254.
12. Lurie B, Van Rysselberghe N, Pennock AT, Upasani VV. Functional outcomes of tillaux and triplane fractures with 2 to 5 millimeters of intra-articular gap. *J Bone Joint Surg Am*. 2020;102(8):679–686.

FOOSHING through the Snow . . .

David Fernandez, Bindu N. Setty, and Isabel A. Barata

Case Study

A 6-year-old boy presents to the Emergency Department (ED) with right elbow pain and refusal to move his arm. The father said he was playing in the park with his older brother on the monkey bars, when he slipped and fell onto his right arm. The fall was witnessed by the father, who denies any head trauma or loss of consciousness. Patient immediately began to cry and clutched his right elbow. When asked where the pain is, the boy points to his elbow. He denies any numbness or tingling sensation and can wiggle his fingers. His heart rate is 101 beats per minute, respiratory rate is 16 breaths per minute, and blood pressure is 102/63mmHg.

Examination is notable for intact skin, flexed elbow, and adducted arm. There is swelling over the right elbow and range of motion limited due to pain. Intrinsic hand muscles are intact, radial pulse 2 + bilaterally, capillary refill <2 seconds, and sensation is intact.

What do you do now?

DISCUSSION

There is compelling evidence in this case that suggests this patient has a fracture of the elbow.

The differential diagnosis includes supracondylar fracture, lateral condyle fracture, medial epicondyle fracture, olecranon fracture, and elbow dislocation. The most common pediatric elbow fractures are supracondylar fractures, lateral condyle fractures, and medial epicondyle fractures. The mechanism of injury between the three is similar and the presentation is nearly identical. Olecranon fractures, however, are uncommon and can be associated with osteogenesis imperfecta (OI). It is necessary to gather history of genetic abnormalities and previous fractures, and to take note of physical exam findings consistent with OI, such as blue sclera and ligamentous laxity.

Given the differentials, radiographs are required, and the recommended views are anteroposterior (AP) and lateral x-rays of the elbow. Knowledge of the anatomy of the elbow is also important, as the age of ossification and age of fusion are two independent events that must be differentiated.

Ossification Center	Years at Ossification	Years at Fusion
Capitellum	1	12
Radial head	4	15
Medial epicondyle	6	17
Trochlea	8	12
Olecranon	10	15
Lateral epicondyle	12	12

The typical patient with a supracondylar fracture is a child between the ages of 5–7 years who falls on an outstretched arm. The hallmark feature is elbow pain and refusal to move the elbow. It is important to perform a neurovascular exam prior to performing any manipulation or reduction maneuvers to be certain that there are no nerve or vascular injuries present. It is important to evaluate for anterior interosseous nerve (AIN) neuropraxia, the inability to flex the interphalangeal joint of the thumb and the distal interphalangeal joint of the index finger. This can be accomplished by asking the patient to make the "A-OK sign" with their fingers. Additionally, it is necessary to evaluate for medial and radial nerve injuries as well, by assessing sensation over the volar aspect of the index finger and the ability to extend the wrist, metacarpophalangeal joints (MCP), and thumb interphalangeal joint (IP). Conducting a proper vascular exam is also necessary to evaluate for any injury. This can be accomplished by assessing for palpable pulses and assessing vascular perfusion.

DIAGNOSIS

The first step to an accurate diagnosis is an adequately obtained orthogonal views of the elbow joint.

The anteroposterior view should be performed with the elbow in full extension and the forearm supinated. For the lateral projection, the elbow should be flexed 90 degrees with the forearm in supination. Both the humerus and forearm should be in full contact with the table on which the cassette rests. The cassette should be well centered about the elbow joint, and the long axis of the cassette should be parallel to that of the forearm. Acquiring a true orthogonal lateral view is crucial. To obtain an optimal lateral view, the posterior supracondylar ridges of the humerus are superimposed, the radial tuberosity is oriented anteriorly, the radial head and coronoid process are partially superimposed, and the olecranon process is viewed in profile.

The radiographs are then interrogated for the presence or absence of an elbow effusion. Traditionally, the presence of an elbow effusion on a 2-view radiograph without an obvious lucency is suspicious for an occult fracture. The specificity ranges from 54% to 90%, as reported by several authors.

The anterior humeral line and the radial head capitellar line are used to assess for alignment of the elbow (Figures 13.1a and 13.1b). On the lateral radiograph, a line drawn along the anterior humeral cortex should bisect the middle third of the capitellum in a child older than 2.5 years. In younger children, the anterior humeral line may intersect the anterior third of the capitellum. For all children, a line parallel to and bisecting the radial head and neck should intersect with the capitellum on all projections. If

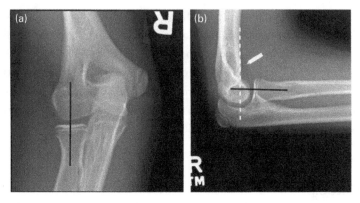

FIGURES 13.1a AND 13.1b. Frontal (a) and lateral (b) views of a normal right elbow in a 12-year-old. A normal anterior fat pad is seen on Figure 13.1b (arrow). Note normal radial head capitellar line (black line in 13.1a and 13.1b). Note normal anterior humeral line (dashed line on 13.1b).

the integrity of one or both of these lines is compromised, then fracture or dislocation, or both, should be suspected.

The fat pad sign is a reliable marker for elbow joint effusion and raises suspicion for fracture in the setting of trauma. The posterior humeral fat pad is situated in the intercondylar depression of the distal humerus and is not visible on a normal lateral elbow radiograph. The anterior humeral fat pad is normally visible on a well-positioned lateral view as a thin lucent arc anterior to the distal humerus (Figure 13.1b). When a joint effusion is present, the posterior fat pad is displaced out of its fossa by fluid and becomes visible on the lateral image (Figure 13.2). The anterior fat pad also gets displaced and becomes more bulbous or sail-like in configuration.

Classification of Supracondylar Fractures

Type 1

Nondisplaced fractures, where the anterior humeral line still bisects the capitellum and the olecranon fossa remains intact (Figures 13.3a and 13.3b).

Type 2

The primary distal fragment is displaced posteriorly but retains its posterior cortex, which functions as a hinge (Figures 13.4a and 13.4b).

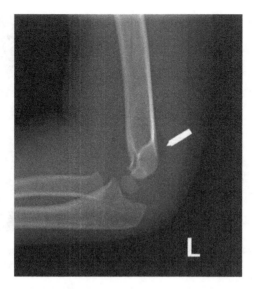

FIGURE 13.2. Lateral view of the elbow in a patient with trauma demonstrates the elevation and visualization of posterior fat pad (arrow) consistent with elbow joint effusion.

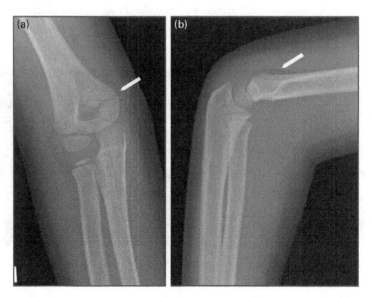

FIGURES 13.3a AND 13.3b. Gartland type I supracondylar fracture (arrow in 13.3a) with no displacement. Note elevated fat pad (arrow in 13.3b).

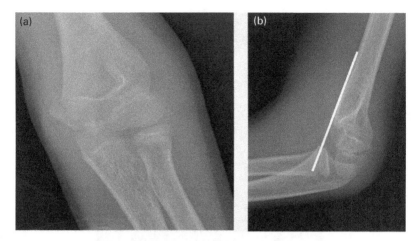

FIGURES 13.4a AND 13.4b. Gartland type II supracondylar fracture where the primary distal fragment is displaced posteriorly but retains its posterior cortex. Note abnormal anterior humeral line (line on 13.4b).

Type 3

Circumferential cortical breach with the distal fragment displaced posteriorly (Figures 13.5a–c).

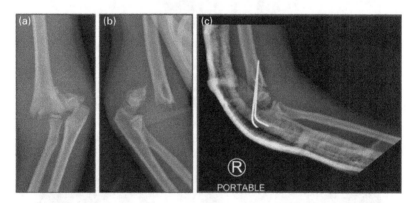

FIGURE 13.5a, 13.5b, AND 13.5c. Gartland type III supracondylar fracture with displaced distal fragment (13.5a and 13.5b). Figure 13.5c demonstrates percutaneous pinning to reduce the fracture.

Grading of Fractures Diagnosed by Gartland Classification

Fracture Type	Characteristics	Comments
I	Minimal displacement	Fat pad elevation on radiographs
II	Posterior hinge	Anterior humeral line anterior to capitellum
III	Displaced	No cortical contact
IV	Displaced in extension and flexion	Flexion and extension instability demonstrated radiographically
Medial comminution	Collapse of medial column	Loss of Baumann's angle*

* Baumann's angle is used for assessing supracondylar fractures (distal fracture of the humerus).

- The angle is determined by drawing a line straight down through the middle of the humeral shaft and then through the trochlea and then drawing a line that is perpendicular to the humeral shaft line. Then a line is made parallel, but running through the lateral condylar physis.
- The angle between the humeral shaft line and the parallel line to the lateral condylar physis should be about 70–75 degrees.

TREATMENT

Treatment is either nonoperative or operative, depending on the displacement of the injury. Nonoperative treatment consists of a long arm cast with less than 90 degrees of elbow flexion. Patients are typically in the cast for approximately 3–4 weeks and require repeat radiographs at week 1 to assess for interval displacement. Operative treatment is done via closed or open reduction with percutaneous pinning and is utilized in patients with severe displacement and neurovascular compromise.

One of the complications of supracondylar fractures is fracture malunion, which can lead to valgus or varus deformities. Malunion may also occur because of pin migration during operative treatment. As with all intervention, infection is a complication but is typically superficial and can be treated with oral antibiotics. Volkmann ischemic contracture is a rare, but serious complication that may result from elbow hyperflexion during casting. The hyperflexion causes an increase in the deep volar forearm compartment pressure and the subsequent loss of radial pulse.

CASE CONCLUSION

The radiographs of the child show a posterior fat pad, type I Gartland fracture. The patient is placed in a posterior splint and followed up by orthopedics for casting. Fracture is completely healed in 4 weeks and the child's cast is removed.

KEY POINTS

- Supracondylar fractures are the most common traumatic fractures seen in the pediatric population and typically occur in children 5–7 years of age from a fall on an outstretched hand with the elbow in extension.
- Proper and thorough physical exam is needed to evaluate for neurovascular injury.
- Management is dependent on the degree of displacement and presence of neurovascular injury.

TIPS FROM THE RADIOLOGIST

- Diagnosis is made by adequately obtained AP and lateral radiographs of the elbow.
- Look for normal orientation of the anterior humeral line intersecting the middle third of the capitellum and a normal radial head capitellar line intersecting the capitellum and radial head on normal AP and lateral elbow radiographs.

- Visualization of distal humeral posterior fat pad and elevation of the anterior fat pad suggests elbow joint effusion that raises suspicion for radiographically occult fracture.
- Gartland classification is used to classify supracondylar distal humeral fractures.

Further Reading

1. Ballinger PW. *Merrill's Atlas of Radiographic Positions and Radiologic Procedures*. 8th ed. St Louis, MO: Mosby, 1995:102–103.

2. Iyer RS, Thapa MM, Khanna PC, Chew FS. Pediatric bone imaging: imaging elbow trauma in children--a review of acute and chronic injuries. *AJR Am J Roentgenol*. 2012 May;198(5):1053–1068. doi: 10.2214/AJR.10.7314. PMID: 22528894.

3. Rogers LF, Malave S, White H, et al. Plastic bowing, torus and greenstick supracondylar fractures of the humerus: radiographic clues to obscure fractures of the elbow in children. *Radiology*. 1978;128:145–150.

4. Jacoby SM, Herman MJ, Morrison WB, Osterman AL. Pediatric elbow trauma: an orthopaedic perspective on the importance of radiographic interpretation. *Semin Musculoskelet Radiol*. 2007;11:48–56.

5. Norell H-G. Roentgenologic visualization of extracapsular fat. *Acta Radiol*. 1954;42:205–210.

6. Gartland JJ. Management of supracondylar fractures of the humerus in children. *Surg Gynecol Obstet*. 1959 Aug;109(2):145–154. PMID: 13675986.

7. Mallo G, Stanat SJ, Ganney J. Use of the Gartland classification system for treatment of pediatric supracondylar humerus fractures. *Orthopedics*. 2010;33:19.

8. Omid R, Choi PD, Skaggs DL. Supracondylar humeral fractures in children. *J Bone Joint Surg Am J*. 2008;90(5):1121–1132. doi:10.2106/JBJS.G.01354.

9. Alton TB, Werner SE, Gee AO. Classifications in brief: the Gartland classification of supracondylar humerus fractures. *Clin Orthop Relat Res*. 2015 Feb;473(2):738–741. doi: 10.1007/s11999-014-4033-8. Epub 2014 Nov 1. PMID: 25361847; PMCID: PMC4294919.

10. Hill CE, Cooke S. Common paediatric elbow injuries. *Open Orthop J*. 2017 Nov 30;11:1380–1393. doi: 10.2174/1874325001711011380. PMID: 29290878; PMCID: PMC5721346.

11. Hohloch L, Eberbach H, Wagner FC, Strohm PC, Reising K, Südkamp NP, Zwingmann J. Age- and severity-adjusted treatment of proximal humerus fractures in children and adolescents-A systematical review and meta-analysis. *PLoS One*. 2017 Aug 24;12(8):e0183157. doi: 10.1371/journal.pone.0183157. PMID: 28837601; PMCID: PMC5570290.

12. Mallo G, Stanat SJ, Ganney J. Use of the Gartland classification system for treatment of pediatric supracondylar humerus fractures. *Orthopedics*. 2010;33:19.
13. Vaquero-Picado A, González-Morán G, Moraleda L. Management of supracondylar fractures of the humerus in children. *EFORT Open Rev*. 2018 Oct 1;3(10):526–540. doi: 10.1302/2058-5241.3.170049. PMID: 30662761; PMCID: PMC6335593.

14 Sentinel Injuries: It's What's Inside That Counts

Madeline Zito, Summit Shah, Isabel A. Barata, and Dana Kaplan

Case Study

A 4-month-old male is brought into the Emergency Department (ED) by his mother, who is concerned that the child has not been moving his right leg after falling off the bed earlier that day. The fall was witnessed by the mother and she immediately brought him to the ED for evaluation. Vital signs are normal for age. Physical exam shows a developmentally appropriate 4-month-old who is moving all of his extremities except for the right leg. No erythema, bruising, or edema is noted on the leg and distal pulses are intact. There are no bruises, lesions, or rashes noted on a thorough skin examination. X-ray of the involved extremity showed a fracture of the distal tibia (Figure 14.1).

What do you do now?

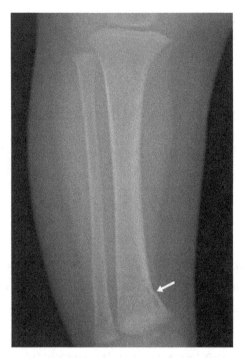

FIGURE 14.1. Right lower extremity radiograph shows cortical break and irregularity (arrow) at the medial aspect of the right distal tibia compatible with acute fracture. No signs of healing.

DISCUSSION

Fractures are the second most common injury occurring as a result of child physical abuse. While accidental fractures frequently occur in ambulatory children, abusive fractures usually occur in non-ambulatory children. With normal development, a child begins to "cruise" at approximately 9 months of age, and begins walking anywhere from 12 to 15 months of age. Approximately 80% of abusive fractures occur in those less than 18 months of age, while only 2% of accidental fractures are found in this age group.[1] Although a child's age is an important risk factor for abusive fractures, other pieces of the history and physical exam, such as the presence of multiple fractures, fractures in different ages or stages of healing, parental delay in seeking medical attention, the existence of other highly suspicious injuries, and an implausible history are suggestive of an abusive etiology.[2]

Being familiar with the loading patterns and forces required to fracture bone can help physicians determine if the history provided matches the mechanism of injury. Transverse fractures are a result of perpendicular forces on the bone that bends it, such as a direct blow; torus or buckle fractures are due to axial loading or compressive forces transmitted down the long axis of the bone; spiral fractures reflect torsional forces due to twisting; oblique fractures represent a combination of bending and twisting forces.[1]

There is no fracture without the potential to be abusive; however, some fractures are more commonly seen in cases of child physical abuse than others. Fractures with a high association with abuse include classic metaphyseal lesions (CMLs), rib fractures, scapular fractures, spinous process fractures, and sternal fractures. Fractures with moderate association with abuse are multiple, bilateral fractures, fractures of different ages, epiphyseal separations, vertebral body fractures and subluxations, digital fractures, and complex skull fractures. Fractures with a low association with child physical abuse are clavicular fractures, subperiosteal new bone formation, long-bone shaft fractures, and linear skull fractures.[2] Regardless of high, moderate, and low association, providers should not rely on this fracture stratification rating to guide their management of patients, but should take it into consideration along with the patient's full history and physical exam.

Despite long bone shaft fractures falling into the low association category, single long bone diaphyseal fractures are the most common fracture pattern identified in abused children, specifically fractures of the femur, humerus, and tibia.[2] A tibial fracture is the third most common extremity injury in abused children, and this is the type of fracture sustained by the patient in our vignette. Most inflicted tibial fractures occur in the distal metaphysis and are initially seen along the medial aspect of the metaphysis, with extension into the lateral metaphysis with more extensive injuries.[1] Our patient is 4 months old, and thus developmentally non-ambulatory, presenting with a fracture of the distal tibia. Despite the history of a traumatic fall off the bed, the presence of a fracture in a non-ambulatory patient warrants a further workup to evaluate for physical abuse.

Furthermore, the distal tibia fracture sustained by our patient should be classified as a sentinel injury. Sentinel injuries are seemingly minor and benign medical injuries that can be indicative of physical abuse. They can even be as simple as a singular bruise on a non-ambulatory infant. A core attribute of a sentinel injury is that it should prompt the physician to consider a diagnosis of physical abuse and lead them to pursue a further workup for additional occult injuries, including a skeletal survey, neuroimaging, liver function tests, and retinal exam.[3] One study which aimed to determine the rates of abuse evaluation and diagnosis among children with commonly considered sentinel injuries showed that the top four sentinel injuries associated with a confirmed abuse diagnosis were rib fractures (56.1%), intracranial hemorrhage (26.3%), abdominal trauma (24.5%), and radius/ulna/tibia/fibula fracture (19.2%).[4] Another study found that 27.5% of definitely abused infants had a previous sentinel injury, and the most common sentinel injuries in the definitely abused population were bruises (80%).[5] It is very important to pick up on sentinel injuries, as missing them puts the child at risk for continuing, even more serious abuse, and possibly death.

While there is a history of possible trauma in our case, more information as to the specifics of the fall are required; the height of the fall, the surface onto which the child fell are two examples. The mere presence of a fracture or other injury in a non-ambulatory patient, especially if they are less than 6 months of age, should prompt a workup for child physical abuse.

WHAT DO YOU DO NOW?

The first step is classifying our distal tibial fracture as a sentinel injury in a non-mobile 4-month-old; the next steps include prompt neuroimaging, laboratory work (including liver function tests), and a skeletal survey, with additional considerations of an ophthalmologic exam. Given that intracranial hemorrhage has higher morbidity and mortality than fractures seen on skeletal survey, it is more prudent and time efficient, especially in the ED setting, to obtain neuroimaging first.

Abusive head trauma (AHT) is the number one cause of fatal child physical abuse in young children, thus something clinicians do not want to miss, as delays in detection and treatment lead to increasing morbidity and mortality. Abusive head trauma, formerly known as "shaken baby syndrome," is an all-encompassing diagnosis, recognizing that the injury mechanism is multifactorial, including shaking alone, impact alone, or both shaking and impact. Additionally, the diagnosis may include multiple components such as a subdural hematoma, intracranial and spinal changes, complex retinal hemorrhages, and fractures that are highly suspicious for abuse.[6]

Deciding whether or not to obtain head imaging in cases of potential abuse can be challenging. When a child presents with altered mental status, seizures, scalp swelling, or other signs of potential head injury, head imaging is routinely performed. However, children, more notably infants, can have clinically significant head injuries that are not detected in the history or during physical examination. Since they are less likely to present with obvious symptoms suggestive of head injury, the decision to evaluate for occult head injuries warrants more careful consideration, as there are risks of neuroimaging. The risk of radiation exposure from computed tomography (CT) scan and the risk of sedation associated with magnetic resonance imaging (MRI) must be weighed against the possibility of missing a head injury. One study which aimed to quantify the yield of head imaging to identify occult head injuries in infants with concern for physical abuse found that while only 1% of infants less than 12 months were found to have occult head injuries, 9.7% of infants less than 6 months were found to have occult head injuries. These findings led them to recommend that infants less than 6 months of age are at the highest risk for occult head injury and should be imaged when presenting with other injuries that raise concern for physical abuse.[7]

The American College of Radiology (ACR) recommends a CT of the head without contrast to evaluate children of all ages for suspected abusive head trauma, especially those found to have complex skull fractures or multiple fractures, children with neurologic changes or apnea, and children with facial injuries raising concern for abuse. A CT of the head is not for general screening. Although there is no strong evidence to recommend universal screening with neuroimaging, clinicians should have a very low threshold for performing head imaging in young children less than 24 months of age with suspected child abuse, as the neurologic exam is less reliable for pathology, and age is an important predictive factor of AHT. In contrast, in older children, greater than 24 months of age, where the neurologic exam is more reliable for detecting intracranial injuries, and when there is low suspicion for AHT, there is less utility in imaging.[3]

Another head imaging modality to consider is an MRI of the head without contrast. MRI is sensitive for the detection of small volume extra-axial hemorrhage and for brain parenchymal injury, which are not evident on CT scan. Furthermore, MRI is sensitive for detecting diffuse axonal injury and microhemorrhages, and can provide prognostic information in AHT. MRI is more appropriate in the non-emergent setting, as it is a lengthy scan and often requires the child to be sedated.[3] Taking into consideration the ACR recommendations, along with the age of our patient, and the findings of a fracture of the distal tibia, a head CT without contrast is the next step (Figures 14.2a and 14.2b).

The most commonly observed intracranial lesions in infants with abusive head trauma are subdural hematomas (SDH) that cover large surface areas of the brain.[7] They are much more common in non-accidental than accidental injuries in infants. SDH in abusive head trauma occurs secondary to tears in the bridging veins that cross the subdural space. These tears are the result of inertial forces. Inertial forces result from the abrupt acceleration/deceleration of the internal tissues within the skull. This is in contrast to contact or impact forces that occur when an immobilized head is struck against an object or a surface, causing damage at the site of the impact/contact.[1]

When dealing with SDH in the setting of AHT, ophthalmologic injury must always be considered, with retinal hemorrhages being the most common ophthalmologic manifestation. Retinal hemorrhages are seen in approximately 75% of children with AHT. Any child with visible eye injury, unexplained altered mental status, or intracranial hemorrhage should be seen by ophthalmology. With AHT, the absence of external eye injury does not rule out retinal hemorrhages. The exam should occur within the first 24 hours of presentation, or at least within 72 hours, as retinal hemorrhages have the potential to heal quickly. Examination findings of multiple ("too numerous to count"), bilateral, and multilayered retinal hemorrhages that extend to the periphery of the retina are highly specific for AHT. Ophthalmologic examination is neither a screening tool, nor a substitution for brain imaging, in cases of children with AHT having normal neurologic exams.[8]

The next component of the workup is a complete skeletal survey, which is recommended for any patient under 24 months of age where there is a suspicion for child physical abuse. The radiographic skeletal survey is used to detect clinically silent fractures, both acute and healing, in children less

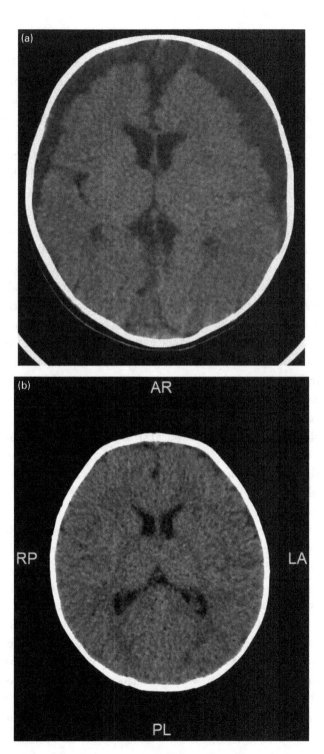

FIGURES 14.2 AND 14.2B. (a) Non-contrast head CT shows bilateral subdural collections overlying the cerebral convexities. There is mass effect with slight rightward midline shift. (b) For comparison, a normal head CT in a different 4-month-old without extra axial collections or midline shift.

than 24 months of age. According to the American College of Radiology, the skeletal survey consists of 21 dedicated views, including front and lateral views of the skull, lateral views of the cervical spine and thoracolumbar spine, and single frontal views of the long bones, hands, feet, chest, and abdomen, and oblique views of the ribs.[3] It is also recommended to repeat the skeletal survey 2 weeks after the initial presentation when abnormal or equivocal findings are found on the initial imaging study and when abuse is clinically suspected, in order to assess for healing fractures that were not seen in their acute phase on the initial skeletal survey. To reduce the child's radiation exposure, the films of the pelvis, spine, and skull can be omitted if there were no concerns in these areas on initial skeletal survey.[3] A "babygram," which is a single x-ray of the entire infant, is diagnostically inadequate and must never be substituted for a complete skeletal survey.[1] In some instances where bone injury is considered to be occult, equivocal, or subtle on plain films, bone scintigraphy can be conducted as an adjunct to skeletal survey. Limitations include injuries near the growth plates where there is a normally increased bone activity, and the study requires venipuncture for radiotracer introduction and often sedation.[3] Figure 14.3 and Figure 14.4 represent two images with significant findings from the full 21-image skeletal survey.

Classic metaphyseal lesions (CMLs) are a series of microfractures through the primary spongiosa of the metaphysis, the most immature portion of the bone. The most common sites for CMLs are the proximal tibia, the distal femur, and the proximal humerus. They are a result of complex forces in the setting of violently shaking an infant, causing flailing of the extremities, or violent traction and twisting of an extremity. Rapid acceleration and deceleration deliver forces through the primary spongiosa causing trabecular bone separation, the point of fracture. These forces are not common in accidental situations, and thus CMLs are highly suspicious for abuse in infancy and are generally only described in children less than 1 year of age. CMLs can have the appearance of a corner or a bucket-handle fracture, depending on the x-ray projection, anteroposterior or lateral. Acute CMLs can be difficult to see on x-rays and commonly heal without subperiosteal new bone formation or marginal sclerosis, thus making them difficult to detect in the healing phases. CMLs are the most common long bone fracture found in fatal infant abuse cases. Thus, much

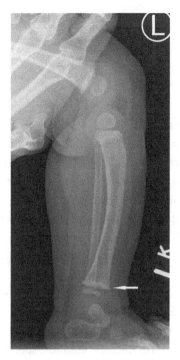

FIGURE 14.3. Left lower extremity radiograph shows metaphyseal corner fracture at the anterior distal aspect of the left tibia (arrow).

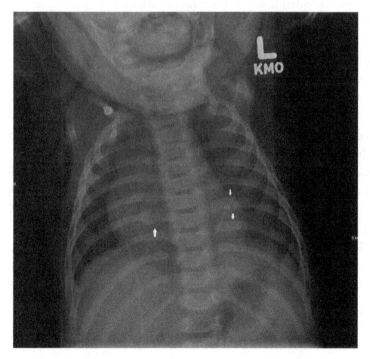

FIGURE 14.4. Chest radiograph shows subacute healing bilateral posterior medial rib fractures involving the right 8th rib and left 8th and 9th ribs (arrows).

diligence is required to identify this type of injury early in order to prevent more severe abuse and even death.[1,2]

Rib fractures are considered highly suspicious for non-accidental trauma. One study showed that the positive predictive value of rib fractures for abuse was 100% in infants younger than 2 years of age and 95% in children younger than 3 years of age.[9] Rib fractures are uncommon in the setting of minor trauma in healthy infants and children. The immature thoracic cage does not easily allow for fractures as it is relatively compliant and mobile, unless subjected to extremely high forces, like one would see in a high-speed motor vehicle crash.[1] Other less common causes of rib fractures in infants are significant trauma sustained during a difficult childbirth, or minor trauma in infants with underlying conditions causing bone fragility.[2]

The proposed mechanism by which rib fractures occur in the context of AHT is when the infant is held with the chest wall in compression. This creates a lever of the proximal rib over the fulcrum of the transverse process, causing a posterior rib fracture, the most specific type of rib fracture suggesting child physical abuse. Fractures can also be seen laterally along the posterior arc of the rib as these compressive forces increase. Anterior and costochondral junction fractures are difficult to detect on x-ray and thus are often underreported. In general, rib fractures are usually multiple and bilateral, as the thoracic cage absorbs and equally distributes the forces applied.[1]

Acute, non-displaced rib fractures can be difficult to see on x-ray. Asymmetry in the appearance of the ribs at the costovertebral junction may be the only radiographic evidence of fracture. Costovertebral fractures may only appear as a small expansion of the head and neck of the rib. In addition to the anteroposterior and lateral x-rays, right and left posterior oblique views should be added to help identify any posterior and lateral rib fractures. Healing rib fractures will present with circular appearing callus formation on x-ray, thus repeat imaging can be done in 2 weeks to help determine if there were initial fractures.[1]

Some theorize the possibility of rib fractures as a result of CPR. Conventional CPR with 2 fingers of a single hand rarely causes rib fractures in children. An alternative method of CPR using 2 hands encircling the rib cage has been associated with rib fractures in one small study conducted on post-mortem infants with a history of 2-handed CPR. Researchers found that 2-handed CPR was associated with multiple, sometimes bilateral, anterolateral rib fractures of the 3rd to 6th ribs, uniformly involving the 4th rib. However, no posterior rib fractures were found. Given the differences in rib fracture characteristics between this study and in abuse, more in-depth research is required.[2]

CASE CONCLUSION

To summarize, our patient sustained a fracture of the distal tibia, a sub-dural hematoma, a CML of the distal tibia, and rib fractures, a collection of findings consistent with child physical abuse. He did proceed to have a normal retinal exam and liver function tests with both the AST and ALT less than 80, which is the cutoff for imaging to exclude occult abdominal injury, which is an infrequent cause of child physical abuse but the second most common cause of fatal child physical abuse.[10] A history of trauma may account for a single injury, but without a thorough workup, clinicians can miss the constellation of abusive findings, thus allowing the child to be subjected to further abuse.

KEY POINTS

- Whenever an infant presents with an injury, even if found incidentally, the diagnosis of child physical abuse must always be considered.
- Child abuse can occur in families of any race, religion, or socioeconomic status; thus clinicians must be aware of their own biases.
- Age is one of the most important factors in determining the pursuit of an abuse workup.
- The developmental stage of the child must always be considered when determining the plausibility of a proposed mechanism of injury.

· A history of trauma may account for a single injury, but without a thorough workup clinicians can miss a constellation of abusive findings, allowing the child to be subjected to further abuse.

TIPS FROM THE RADIOLOGIST

· Satisfaction of search: do not fail to continue search for subsequent abnormalities after identifying an initial one.
· Know the high-specificity fractures for child abuse: classic metaphyseal lesions, posterior rib fractures, scapular fractures, spinous processes fractures, sternal fractures.
· Know the low-specificity fractures for child abuse: clavicular fractures, long bone shaft fractures, linear skull fractures.
· If uncertain findings, recommend follow-up imaging to look for healing or new findings.
· A "babygram"/single x-ray of the entire infant is diagnostically inadequate and must never be substituted for a complete skeletal survey.

Further Reading
1. Reece RM, Christian C, eds. *Child Abuse: Medical Diagnosis and Management*. 3rd ed. Elk Grove Village, IL: American Academy of Pediatrics; 2008.
2. Flaherty EG, Perez-Rossello JM, Levine MA, Hennrikus WL; American Academy of Pediatrics Committee on Child Abuse and Neglect; Section on Radiology, American Academy of Pediatrics; Section on Endocrinology, American Academy of Pediatrics; Section on Orthopaedics, American Academy of Pediatrics; Society for Pediatric Radiology. Evaluating children with fractures for child physical abuse. *Pediatrics*. 2014 Feb;133(2):e477–489.
3. Expert Panel on Pediatric Imaging; Wootton-Gorges SL, Soares BP, Alazraki AL, Anupindi SA, Blount JP, Booth TN, Dempsey ME, Falcone RA Jr, Hayes LL, Kulkarni AV, Partap S, Rigsby CK, Ryan ME, Safdar NM, Trout AT, Widmann RF, Karmazyn BK, Palasis S. ACR Appropriateness Criteria® suspected physical abuse-child. *J Am Coll Radiol*. 2017 May;14(5S):S338–S349.
4. Lindberg DM, Beaty B, Juarez-Colunga E, Wood JN, Runyan DK. Testing for abuse in children with sentinel injuries. *Pediatrics*. 2015 Nov;136(5):831–838.
5. Sheets LK, Leach ME, Koszewski IJ, Lessmeier AM, Nugent M, Simpson P. Sentinel injuries in infants evaluated for child physical abuse. *Pediatrics*. 2013 Apr;131(4):701–707.

6. Choudhary AK, Servaes S, Slovis TL, Palusci VJ, Hedlund GL, Narang SK, Moreno JA, Dias MS, Christian CW, Nelson MD Jr, Silvera VM, Palasis S, Raissaki M, Rossi A, Offiah AC. Consensus statement on abusive head trauma in infants and young children. *Pediatr Radiol*. 2018 Aug;48(8):1048–1065.

7. Henry MK, Feudtner C, Fortin K, Lindberg DM, Anderst JD, Berger RP, Wood JN. Occult head injuries in infants evaluated for physical abuse. *Child Abuse Negl*. 2020 May;103:104431.

8. Christian CW, Levin AV; Council on Child Abuse and Neglect; Section on Opthalmology; American Association of Certified Orthoptists; American Association for Pediatric Ophthalmology and Strabismus; American Academy of Ophthalmology. The eye examination in the evaluation of child abuse. *Pediatrics*. 2018 Aug;142(2):e20181411.

9. Barsness KA, Cha E-S, Bensard DD, et al. The positive predictive value of rib fractures as an indicator of nonaccidental trauma in children [see comment]. *J Trauma*. 2003;54(6):1107–1110.

10. Glick JC, Lorand MA, Bilka KR. Physical abuse of children. *Pediatr Rev*. 2016 Apr;37(4):146–156.

15 What a Pain in the Neck

Michael Sperandeo and
Gayathri Sreedher

Case Study

A 6-year-old girl was transported by Emergency Medical Services (EMS) to a Pediatric Level 1 Trauma Center after she was struck on her bicycle by an oncoming vehicle. She was thrown and had a loss of consciousness. She was wearing her helmet, and it appears to be cracked from the accident. A cervical collar was placed by the EMS crew. On arrival at the ED her vital signs are: heart rate 139 bpm, blood pressure 105/65mmHg, respiratory rate 27bpm, temperature 99.2°F, oxygen saturation (SpO2) 99% on room air. Her airway is intact, she has equal bilateral breath sounds, and palpable pulses in all four extremities. Glasgow Coma Scale (GCS) is 14. She complains of neck and back pain and moves all extremities upon command. There are no other obvious bony injuries. Pelvis is stable. You note multiple scattered abrasions and contusions across her face, upper extremities, and lower extremities. When you attempt to roll her, she starts crying. Her exam is limited as she cannot endorse spinal point tenderness, but there are no step-offs.

What do I do now?

INTRODUCTION

Cervical spine injuries are a frightening diagnosis to make for even the most seasoned pediatric emergency medicine physician. Detection of cervical spine injuries in the ED are paramount to prevent permanent disability, poor neurological outcomes, or death. Clinical assessment is frequently very difficult. Often, patients can offer only limited history due to an altered mental status, young age, pain, crying, or other emotional stress. Determining a child's neurological status and assessing for spinal tenderness often requires patience and a strong clinical acumen. Fortunately, cervical spine injuries in the setting of trauma are rare in the pediatric population. However, when a spinal injury does occur in a child, the cervical spine is involved 60%–80% of the time, compared to only 30%–40% in adults.

Anatomical and structural differences predispose younger children to higher-level cervical spine injuries than older children and adults. The pediatric cervical spine remains underdeveloped until about age 8 years. Thereafter, it starts to take on characteristics more consistent with the adult cervical spine. Up until that point, children have a disproportionately larger and heavier skull than adults. This shifts the child's center of gravity cranially, likewise shifting their cervical motion fulcrum-point more superiorly. Combined with an underdeveloped ligamentous and muscle structure, children under 8 years of age are at a significantly increased risk for higher-level ligamentous disruption and are predisposed to subsequent cervical spine injury. In children younger than 2 years of age, axial region injuries were seen in 74% of cervical spine injuries, compared to 53% in children ages 8–15 years.

Similarly, structural and anatomical differences for children with congenital or other structural pathologies may increase a child's susceptibility to a devastating cervical spine injury. These must be considered when evaluating a child with concern for a cervical spine injury. For example, children with Down syndrome are at particularly increased risk given their ligamentous laxity. Likewise, children with Klippel-Feil syndrome, juvenile rheumatoid arthritis, osteogenesis imperfecta, and Larsen syndrome should all be considered particularly high risk.

EMERGENCY DEPARTMENT EVALUATION AND MANAGEMENT

Initial assessment of all pediatric patients with concern for significant trauma follow Advanced Trauma Life Support guidelines, beginning first with a primary survey with particular focus on airway, breathing, circulation, disability, and completely undressing and exposing the patient. Thereafter, a comprehensive secondary survey, including a complete neurological assessment, should follow. All children with suspected cervical spine injury and/or neurological deficits should be promptly placed in a cervical collar and strict cervical spine immobilization procedures should be maintained.

Once the patient has been determined to be stable, additional history taking and more comprehensive evaluation should begin. Cervical spine injuries may be particularly challenging to detect on physical examination alone. Therefore, the emergency physician must always have a high level of suspicion until the patient is fully evaluated. Higher-level spinal injuries may present with abnormal vital signs including, bradycardia, hypotension, alerted or irregular respirations, or in more severe cases, apnea when diaphragmatic innervation is compromised. However, it is important to remember that hypotension in the setting of trauma must be assumed to be due to hemorrhage until proven otherwise. In alert patients, cervical spine injuries will often, but not always, present with midline cervical tenderness on neck examination. More subtle findings such as paraspinal tenderness, muscle spasm, and decreased range of motion should also increase suspicion, but should be assessed in conjunction with the mechanism of injury. A comprehensive neurological exam, including assessment of GCS, fine and gross motor function and sensation in all extremities, reflexes, and assessment of cranial nerves, should also be performed. Detection of subtle neurological deficits may be challenging. The presence of a completely normal neurological exam does not necessarily exclude cervical spine injury in ambulatory, well-appearing patients. In the setting of a high-risk mechanism, one study found that 18% of children with asymptomatic presentations were determined to have a significant injury.

Mechanism of injury and the severity thereof should also be considered during evaluation for all children with concern for cervical spine injury.

Young infants and toddlers are particularly susceptible to whiplash injuries in the setting of motor vehicle injuries, especially when not properly restrained. Increased cervical laxity makes younger children particularly vulnerable to injury in the setting of a significant fall with head trauma. When stratifying by age group, certain mechanisms of injury are more common than others for cervical spine injuries in each age group. For example, motor vehicle accidents and falls are the most common mechanisms in children less than 2 years old. Sports injuries have a higher predominance in children ages 8–15 years. While unfortunate, child abuse does account for a significant number of cervical spine injuries, particularly in younger and more vulnerable populations. The emergency physician should remain vigilant and maintain a high level of suspicion for abuse when the history, physical exam, social or familial factors do not amount to a plausible mechanism to explain clinical findings.

In the adult population, there are multiple well-validated clinical tools that are utilized frequently to determine whether a patient can be cleared clinically from having a significant cervical spine injury, thereby avoiding unnecessary imaging, hospital resources, and radiation exposure. Frequently cited tools include the NEXUS criteria and the Canadian C-Spine Rule. Unfortunately, while likely still useful to identify patients requiring cervical spine imaging, these tools have not been strongly validated externally to *rule out* pediatric patients with cervical spine injury. Some validation studies have shown promise when these decision tools are applied to older children, age 9 years and older. However, despite these studies, the general consensus in the literature advises to not solely use these tools to exclude significant injury. An additional study conducted by the Pediatric Emergency Care Applied Research Network (PECARN) determined that there were 8 clinical features common in pediatric patients with cervical spine injuries. The study population included in this article was exclusive to children under 16 years of age and included children under 2 years old. The presence of one of the following clinical features, common in pediatric patients under 16 years of age with cervical spine injuries, performed with a sensitivity of 98% and a specificity of 26%; neck pain, torticollis, altered mental status, focal neurological deficit, substantial torso injury, conditions predisposing to cervical injury (i.e., Down syndrome, Ehlers-Danlos, cervical arthritis, etc.), high-risk motor vehicle collision, and diving.

IMAGING MODALITIES CONSIDERATIONS

Once the decision is made that imaging is required to evaluate for cervical spinal injury, careful consideration should be made as to which type of imaging is most indicated. Plain films, computed tomography (CT), and magnetic resonance imaging (MRI) each have a role in pediatric cervical spinal injury assessment, but also should be considered in the context of cost, availability, resource utilization, and radiation exposure risk. The Trauma Association of Canada published a cervical spine radiographic assessment algorithm based on expert consensus after an exhaustive literature search and after examining practice guidelines at various pediatric trauma centers across Canada. These algorithms consider the reliability of physical exam, signs of neurological deficit, cooperativeness of patient, and patient age. In summary, in the reliable patient it is recommended to first attempt to clear the cervical spine clinically utilizing the NEXUS criteria, followed by an assessment of the patient's ability to range the neck without pain. If unable to do so, anteroposterior (AP), lateral, and odontoid plain films are indicated, followed by a neurological assessment. If initial studies are abnormal, pursuing a CT C-spine is the next step, with further escalation to MRI in the setting of abnormal prior studies or persisting neurological deficits.

AP and cross-table lateral cervical films have mixed reports for sensitivity and specificity in the literature. One study cited plain films as 79% sensitive for cervical spine injury, with the addition of an odontoid view increasing sensitivity to 94%. Another study concluded that plain films properly detected cervical spinal injuries in 87% of patients with AP and lateral views; in this study the addition of odontoid views did not aid in diagnosis. Yet another study achieved 100% sensitivity, albeit in a small population size. However, it is important to realize that evaluation of the cervical spine is not complete unless it includes the entire cervical spine, including the C7/T1 junction, which may not be included in all films. When complete assessment of the cervical spine is achieved, plain films may be a reasonable screening imaging modality in patients without focal neurological deficits, a normal exam, and with low-risk mechanisms that otherwise fail alternative clinical screening modalities.

Another reasonable approach would be to forgo screening plain films and move directly to CT in cases where there is concern for other significant injury, high-risk mechanism, patient obtundation, or neurological deficits present on initial examination. CT has been reported to be 98% sensitive in detecting bony cervical spine pathologies; however, it does come at an increased radiation exposure risk when compared to plain films. It is therefore crucial for the ordering physician to use CT judiciously and in the appropriate clinical setting.

MRI remains the gold standard for detecting cervical spinal cord injuries. However, it can be costly, time consuming, and resource intensive; requires a cooperative patient and sedation; and may not be readily available at all care centers. In some instances, patients may require transfer to pediatric trauma centers after consultation with the receiving pediatric trauma or spinal specialist.

NORMAL VARIATIONS

Normal Cervical Spine Radiograph

Interpretation of a normal cervical lateral radiograph in trauma begins with evaluation of the alignment. There is a normal slight lordotic curvature of the spine. The anterior vertebral line parallels the anterior border of the vertebral bodies, the posterior vertebral line parallels the posterior border of the vertebral bodies, the spinolaminar line parallels the posterior margin of the spinal canal, and the posterior spinous line parallels the tips of the spinous processes. The normal prevertebral soft tissues measure less than one-third of the vertebral body width to C3 and less than vertebral body width below C3.

Pseudosubluxation

Pseudosubluxation refers to the apparent anterior displacement of C2 over C3 (most common) and C3 over C4 (less common) on a lateral cervical spine radiograph. It represents a normal variant in up to 20% of children, typically seen in children less than 8 years of age, and is secondary to the horizontal orientation of facet joints in young children. On a lateral radiograph it can be identified by drawing a line from the anterior margin of the posterior arch of C1 to the anterior margin of the posterior arch of C3 (aka the Swischuk's line). The anterior margin of the posterior arch of C2 should be within 1.5–2mm of this line. While pseudosubluxation may be more pronounced on the flexion images, it is considered a normal variant and does not warrant any further assessment. See Figure 15.1 a, 15.1b and 15.1c for spinolaminar line in pseudosubluxation (Figure 15.1a), disruption of the spinolaminar line (Figure 15.1b) and a normal spinolaminar line in an older child (Figure 15.1c).

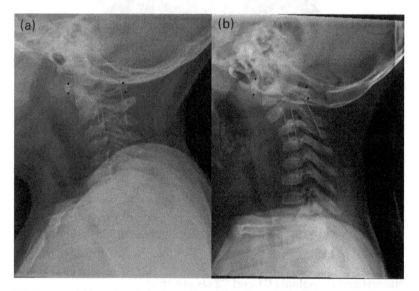

FIGURE 15.1. (a) Lateral cervical spine radiograph in a 15-month-old child, status post-fall, demonstrates C2 over C3 pseudosubluxation. There is less than 25% subluxation and maintained spinolaminar alignment (Swischuk's line). (b) Lateral cervical spine radiograph in a 3-month-old with non-accidental trauma demonstrates disruption of the spinolaminar line and 50% subluxation of C2 over C3. There is also disc space widening at C2/C3 suggestive of ligamentous disruption (seen on MRI later). [C1 anterior and posterior arches are marked by black dots for convenience]. (c) A normal lateral radiograph of the cervical spine for reference in a 7-year-old child. The anterior vertebral line, posterior vertebral line (black line), and the spinolaminar line (white vertical line) are in alignment. The prevertebral space (horizontal white lines) are not widened.

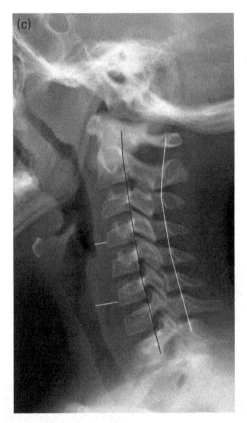

FIGURE 15.1. Continued

PATHOLOGY-SPECIFIC RADIOGRAPHIC FINDINGS, PATTERNS, AND PITFALLS

Normal and Pathologic C1 and C2 Ossification

C1 and C2 ossification centers and their synchondrosis should not be mistaken for fractures in the pediatric age group. Knowledge of the normal centers and their alignment is essential to avoid errors. C2 develops from five ossification centers, the two neural arches, body, odontoid process, and the os terminale (Figure 15.2a demonstrates the normal C2 synchondrosis and Figures 15.2 b–e demonstrate fractures through the synchondroses). Fracture through unfused synchondrosis is an uncommon finding.

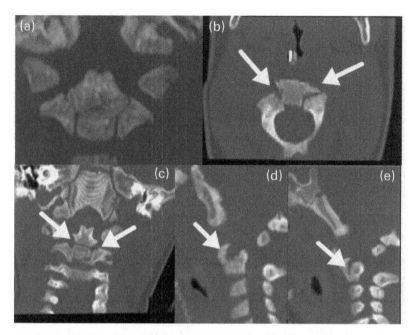

FIGURE 15.2. (a) Coronal CT demonstrates the normal C2 synchondrosis in a 11-month-old child. (b–e) Fractures through synchondroses between the neural arches and the body of C2 and the odontoid process on both sides (right d more than left e) marked by arrows in a 16-month-old child, status post–motor vehicle accident.

Atlanto-axial Rotary Subluxation/Fixation (AARF)

Atlanto-axial rotatory subluxation/fixation includes a spectrum of C1 over C2 subluxation to fixed facet dislocation. Both osseous and ligamentous abnormalities can lead to a fixed rotation of C1 on C2. Higher degrees of rotation may lead to spinal cord compression from canal stenosis. Typical clinical presentation includes "cock robin" head position, from rotation and tilt of the head in relation to C1. Neck pain, headache, and muscular spasm can accompany the torticollis. Radiographs demonstrate asymmetry between the lateral masses of C1 and dens seen on open-mouth view. In severe cases of dislocation there may be increased atlanto-dental interval on lateral cervical spine radiographs. However, when suspected, a three-position CT is the gold standard in imaging. The cervical spine should be imaged from occiput to C2 in presenting position (P), neutral positioning (P0), and with the neck turned to the opposite side (P–) (See Figure 15.3 a,

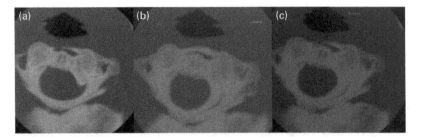

FIGURE 15.3. Three position CT done in presenting (a), neutral (b) and rightward (c) neck rotation demonstrates persistent fixed C1 C2 angulation and loss of normal C1 rotation consistent with atlanto-axial rotatory fixation. The C1 over C2 subluxation is mild in this case. (Maximum intensity projection reformats in 15mm thickness are obtained on a 3D capable workstation.)

b and c). During normal cervical rotation, C1 rotates prior to C2, with C2 rotation lagging behind the initial degrees of rotation. The loss or reduction of this C1 over C2 motion with neck rotation is demonstrated in AARF. The Fielding and Hawkins Classification grades the severity depending on the amount of C1 subluxation over C2. Management is dependent on the degree of severity and should be discussed with neurosurgery. Treatments can range from closed reduction and placement of neck collar to halo traction and, in some persistent cases, open reduction.

Spinal Cord Injury without Radiographic Abnormality (SCIWORA)

A term coined before the advent of widespread use of MRI, SCIWORA is nevertheless an important concept to understand, particularly in the context of children. The presence of spinal cord injury, as evidenced by focal neurological deficits in the absence of a discernible fracture on radiographs and absence of obstetric complications, congenital anomalies, electric shock, and penetrating trauma, forms the basis of SCIWORA. Unfortunately, there is no consensus regarding a unifying definition. Common modes of injury include motor vehicle accidents, nonaccidental trauma, and sports-related injuries. The neurological deficit can stem from a myriad of factors, including ligamentous disruption, disc herniation, and epidural hematoma, among others. Subsequent injury leads to cord infarction, cord edema and/or cord contusion. SCIWORA is more common in the pediatric cervical

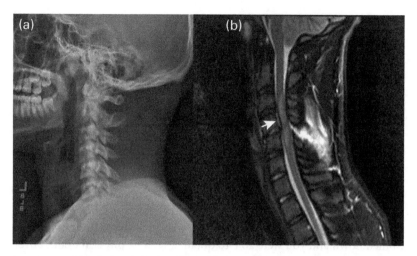

FIGURE 15.4. (a) Sagittal cervical spine radiograph in a 16-year-old with injury during wrestling. Normal radiograph without prevertebral swelling, fracture, or malalignment. Patient has no sensation below the nipple line and quadriplegia. (b) MRI with sagittal STIR Sequence demonstrates cord edema from C3 to C5 with C4/C5 posterior spinal distraction, ligamentous injury, and edema. There is an anterior subligamentous edema opposite C4 further narrowing the canal (arrow).

spine due to ligamentous laxity. MRI is the best imaging modality and demonstrates the etiology as well as extent of spinal cord injury. Figure 15.4 a and b demonstrate a normal lateral cervical spine radiograph with an abnormal MRI.

DISPOSITION

When clinical suspicion remains high or neurological deficits persist, the benefits of transfer, resource utilization, and cost to obtain the most definitive study and specialist evaluation outweigh the risk of missing a clinically important and potentially devastating cervical spine injury. In all cases, cervical spine precautions and/or use of a cervical collar should be maintained until clearance of the cervical spine can be made clinically in a reliable patient or until sufficient radiological evidence has excluded injury.

Patients who can be considered candidates for discharge from the ED are those with low-risk mechanisms, no focal neurological deficits on exam, reassuring and reliable clinical reassessments, and no fractures on imaging.

In addition, availability for close pediatric and/or specialist follow-up and parent/patient comfort should also be considered with regard to disposition. In equivocal cases or where the diagnosis remains unclear, it is recommended and reasonable to escalate and obtain more advanced imaging and specialist evaluation.

CASE CONCLUSION

During the primary survey it was difficult to obtain a reliable physical exam. Evaluation of spinal tenderness and neurological deficits were limited. As such, a cervical collar was placed.

Analgesia was given and after a period of brief observation the patient calmed down and you were able to obtain a reliable physical exam. Given the mechanism, you ordered screening plain films of the cervical spine that did not demonstrate acute pathology. Shortly afterward, the parents inform you that the patient is much calmer, and is now pain free. After a comprehensive neurological exam you appreciate no deficits and there is no spinal tenderness. The collar is removed and the patient is able to range her neck without pain. She is given juice and fruit and is able to tolerate oral fluids. Parents report that she is now acting like her normal self and that they are comfortable with a plan for discharge and close follow-up with the pediatrician tomorrow. They appreciate your close attention to their daughter and your judicious use of imaging and frequent clinical reassessments.

KEY POINTS

- Missing a cervical spine injury can lead to significant morbidity and mortality.
- Traumatic cervical spine injuries are rare in the pediatric patient.
- When injuries occur, they tend to be higher-level cervical spine injuries.
- Cervical spine precautions should be maintained until cervical spine injury is excluded.

- Clinical assessment tools commonly used in adults to clear the cervical spine without imaging have not been validated in pediatric populations.
- In any case of diagnostic uncertainty, concerning physical exam, or abnormal vital signs, once determined stable, prompt transfer or consultation with the appropriate specialist should be arranged.

TIPS FROM THE RADIOLOGIST

- Plain films can be considered for screening in low-risk mechanisms and a reassuring physical exam.
- On cervical radiographs, look for normal alignment of the cervical spine, including the anterior and posterior vertebral body line, the spinolaminar line, and the spinous process line. Look for secondary signs such as prevertebral soft tissue swelling. Normal ossification centers may be inappropriately mistaken for pathologic fractures.
- Three-position CT is necessary to diagnose atlanto-axial rotary fixation.
- MRI remains the gold standard for the exclusion of spinal cord injuries.

Further Reading

1. Baker C, Kadish H, Schunk JE. Evaluation of pediatric cervical spine injuries. *Am J Emerg Med*. 1999;17(3):230–234.
2. Booth TN. Cervical spine evaluation in pediatric trauma. *AJR Am J Roentgenol*. 2012 May;198(5):W417–425. doi: 10.2214/AJR.11.8150.
3. Chung S, Mikrogianakis A, Wales PW, et al. Trauma association of Canada Pediatric Subcommittee National Pediatric Cervical Spine Evaluation Pathway: consensus guidelines. *J Trauma*. 2011;70(4):873–884.
4. Corcoran B, Linscott LL, Leach JL, Vadivelu S. Application of normative occipital condyle-C1 interval measurements to detect atlanto-occipital injury in children. *AJNR Am J Neuroradiol*. 2016 May;37(5):958–962.
5. Cui LW, Probst MA, Hoffman JR, Mower WR. Sensitivity of plain radiography for pediatric cervical spine injury. *Emerg Radiol*. 2016 Oct;23(5):443–448.

6. Gopinathan N, Viswanathan V, Crawford A. Cervical spine evaluation in pediatric trauma: a review and an update of current concepts. *Indian J Orthop*. 2018;52(5):489–500.

7. Hoffman R, Mower WR, Wolfson AB, et al. Validity of a set of clinical criteria to rule out injury to the cervical spine in patients with blunt trauma. *N Engl J Med*. 2000;343(2):94–99.

8. Kos N, Aboudiab M, Atanelov Z, Hathcock A. Cervical spine injuries in the pediatric population. *EMRA*. https://www.emra.org/emresident/article/pediatric-c-spine. Published August 17, 2020. Accessed March 29, 2021.

9. Leonard JC, Kuppermann N, Olsen C, et al. Factors associated with cervical spine injury in children after blunt trauma. *Ann Emerg Med*. 2011;58(2):145–155.

10. Leonard JR, Jaffe DM, Kuppermann N, Olsen CS, Leonard JC; Pediatric Emergency Care Applied Research Network (PECARN) Cervical Spine Study Group. Cervical spine injury patterns in children. *Pediatrics*. 2014;133(5):e1179–1188.

11. Mahajan P, Jaffe DM, Olsen CS, et al. Spinal cord injury without radiologic abnormality in children imaged with magnetic resonance imaging. *J Trauma Acute Care Surg*. 2013;75(5):843–847.

12. McAllister AS, Nagaraj U, Radhakrishnan R. Emergent imaging of pediatric cervical spine trauma. *RadioGraphics*. 2019;39(4):1126–1142.

13. Pang D. Atlantoaxial rotatory fixation. *Neurosurgery*. 2010 Mar;66(3 Suppl):161–183.

14. Pang D, Wilberger JE Jr. Spinal cord injury without radiographic abnormalities in children. *J Neurosurg*. 1982 Jul;57(1):114–129.

15. Shaw M, Burnett H, Wilson A, Chan O. Pseudosubluxation of C2 on C3 in polytraumatized children: prevalence and significance. *Clin Radiol*. 1999 Jun;54(6):377–380.

16. Rusin JA, Ruess L, Daulton RS. New C2 synchondrosal fracture classification system. *Pediatr Radiol*. 2015;45:872–881.

17. Slaar A, Fockens MM, Wang J, Maas M, Wilson DJ, Goslings JC, Schep NWL, van Rijn RR. Triage tools for detecting cervical spine injury in pediatric trauma patients. *Cochrane Database Syst Rev*. 2017;12. Art. No.: CD011686.

18. Swarm M. Cervical spine imaging in pediatric trauma. *EMRA*. https://www.emra.org/emresident/article/cervical-spine-imaging-in-pediatric-trauma/. Published December 3, 2015. Accessed March 29, 2021.

19. Swischuk LE. Anterior displacement of C2 in children: physiologic or pathologic. *Radiology*. 1977;122 (3):759–763.

20. Viccellio P, Simon H, Pressman BD, et al. A prospective multicenter study of cervical spine injury in children. *Pediatrics*. 2001;108(2).

16 Torticollis in a Child with Down Syndrome

Kristy Williamson and

Rachelle Goldfisher

Case Study

A 7-year-old boy presents to the Pediatric Emergency Department (ED) with a "twisted neck." His parents noticed him holding his head to the side, which has progressively worsened. Today he complained of pain and urinated on himself. There were no reports of injury, recent fever, drooling, or other symptoms.

He has a history of Trisomy 21, a repaired atrioventricular (AV) canal, and mild asthma.

On physical examination, he appears uncomfortable but nontoxic. His vitals are as follows: temperature 37°C, heart rate 112 BPM, blood pressure 90/50mmHg, respiratory rate 18bpm, oxygen saturation of 100%. The physical examination is notable for his chin pointing to the left with his head tilted to the right. The child has point tenderness over C1–C3. Cranial nerves are intact with muscle strength of 5/5 in upper extremities and 4/5 in lower extremities, gross sensation intact, and 3 + patellar reflexes bilaterally.

What do you do now?

DISCUSSION

Any patient with cervical spine tenderness and new weakness or sensory deficits should be emergently evaluated. Immediate cervical spine immobilization in a C-collar should be performed. While the differential is extensive and includes traumatic injury to the cervical spine or spinal cord, infectious etiologies, and central nervous system (CNS) tumors, and our patient's history of Down syndrome narrows the differential diagnosis. Providers should immediately be concerned for atlantoaxial instability with subluxation and obtain emergent imaging. In our patient, a cervical collar is placed, and neurosurgery is consulted. A cervical spine radiograph is performed including anteroposterior (AP) and lateral images (Figures 16.1 and 16.2). An open-mouth view is unable to be performed secondary to patient cooperation. The radiographs demonstrate torticollis and reversal of the normal cervical lordosis. While instability may be

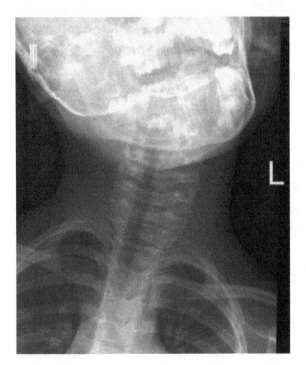

FIGURE 16.1. Anteroposterior (AP) radiograph of the neck demonstrating a leftward tilt of the cervical spine and rightward tilt of the head in keeping with known torticollis.

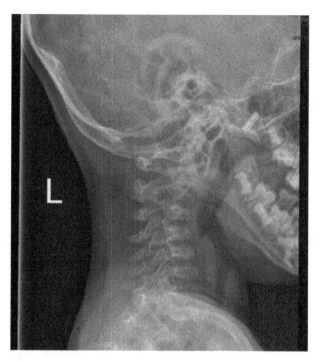

FIGURE 16.2. Lateral radiograph demonstrating reversal of lordosis centered at C3 that may be due to torticollis and patient guarding.

difficult to assess on x-rays without flexion and extension views, providers can rule out an obvious fracture and a retropharyngeal abscess after noting no widening of the prevertebral space. Given the high concern for instability, a computed tomography (CT) scan is obtained (Figure 16.3). The CT demonstrates widening of the interval of the dens and lateral mass of C1 (aka lateral atlantodental interval). Given the obvious instability and neurologic symptoms, the patient was sedated for magnetic resonance imaging (MRI) (Figure 16.4). The MRI demonstrated widening of the anterior atlantodental interval. There is superior migration of the dens and kinking of the cord at the cervical medullary junction. There was no associated signal abnormality within the spinal cord.

Generally, patients with Trisomy 21 are at high risk for numerous orthopedic conditions due to the combination of ligamentous laxity and hypotonia. One of the most feared conditions is atlantoaxial instability, defined

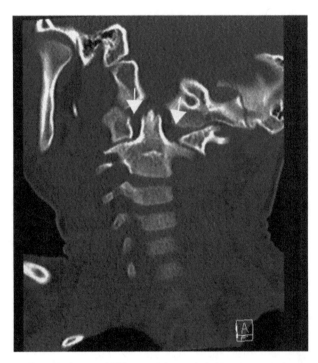

FIGURE 16.3. Coronal reformatted CT image of the cervical spine demonstrating abnormal flexion and rotation of the skull in relation to the C1–C2 vertebra with widening (arrows) of the interval between the dens and lateral mass of C1 without fracture.

as excessive mobility of the articulation of the atlas and the axis due to ligamentous laxity. The instability predisposes patients to subluxation or atlantoaxial rotary subluxation (AARS), which is a rare spectrum of rotational disorders of the atlantoaxial joint that leads to limited rotation of the neck. In some cases, atlantoaxial rotary fixation (AARF) can occur, where the neck remains locked in rotation. In general, AARS may be idiopathic, spontaneous, or traumatic in origin, but children with Trisomy 21 are predisposed due to the known ligamentous laxity. Briefly, the laxity may lead to subluxation of C1 on C2, potentially leading to spinal cord compression.

The atlas (C1) is the most superior cervical vertebra and connects the occiput with the spine. It has masses connected by anterior and posterior arches. The axis (C2) has a dens, or odontoid process, that extends superiorly to articulate with the anterior arch of C1 via the transverse ligament. The

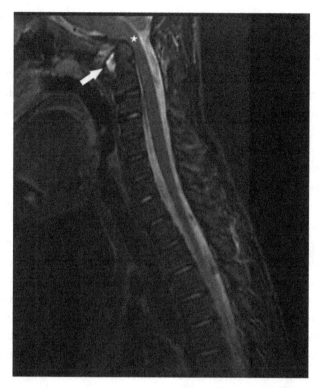

FIGURE 16.4. MRI showing an anterior subluxation of C1 with respect to C2, with widening of the atlanto-dens distance (arrow) and superior migration of the dens. In addition, note kinking (star) of the spinal cord at the cervical medullary junction, but no associated cord signal abnormality.

normal physiologic range of motion of C1 on C2 is 25°–53° to either side. The transverse ligament and paired alar ligaments stabilize the atlantoaxial joint and prevent excessive anterior motion of C1 on C2. Generally, in AARS, the spinal cord is not compromised because the transverse ligament of the atlas remains intact.

It is estimated that 10%–27% of all individuals with Trisomy 21 may have radiological findings of instability, though most are asymptomatic and without subluxation. Only 1%–2% of these patients will develop symptomatic instability, either spontaneously or with even minor trauma. Given this low association of instability and symptomatology, providers must have a high index of suspicion if a patient with Down syndrome presents with any neck pain, torticollis, reduced neck mobility, alteration in gait or clumsiness, deterioration of manipulative skills, or loss of bowel or bladder control. If a patient with Down syndrome presents with any of these findings, further history, a detailed physical exam including full musculoskeletal and neurologic exams, and definite imaging should be performed. Often children with Down syndrome have developmental and intellectual disabilities, making subtle early symptoms difficult to communicate. However, if severe symptoms are not recognized, spinal cord compression can occur suddenly. It has been shown that nearly all of the individuals with Trisomy 21 who experience catastrophic injury to the spinal cord had some preceding neurologic abnormalities, so appropriate screening by providers at all routine and emergency visits should be performed for these children.

Our patient presented with torticollis, which is a lateral twisting of the neck that causes the head to tilt to one side with the chin turned to the opposite side. Acquired torticollis generally can result from sternocleidomastoid or trapezius muscle injury or anterior neck infection, but can also be due to a rotational deformity of the cervical spine. Unlike in adults, non-muscular causes have been implicated in less than <20% of acquired torticollis cases in children. When there is AARS, the head is rotated and flexed, with associated head tilt contralateral to the direction of rotation (in a "cock robin" positioning).

When examining a patient with torticollis, active neck range of motion by the patient should be assessed if there is no numbness or tingling reported. Passive range of motion testing should be performed with caution because of the risk of vertebral subluxation. Providers should assess for direct point tenderness over the cervical spine, which is common in subluxation because of nerve root compression. A thorough neurologic examination should be performed, testing for muscle strength and sensory deficits; motor system abnormalities are the most common presenting symptoms. Patients may have hyperreflexia, the presence of a Babinski sign, or clonus indicative of corticospinal tract involvement. Clinicians can also evaluate for Hoffmann's sign, which involves loosely holding the middle finger and flicking the fingernail downward. A positive sign occurs if there is flexion and adduction of the thumb on the same hand, indicating an upper motor neuron lesion due to cervical cord compression. In severe compression, patients may have quadriparesis or quadriplegia.

Initial management of these children always first involves the "A, B, Cs," or focusing on airway management, breathing, and circulation. If for any reason the child needs to be intubated, a separate provider must always maintain in-line immobilization of the cervical spine. In general, for any child presenting with neck pain, a C-collar should be immediately placed in triage. Of note, the neck should not be corrected to midline when the cervical collar is placed if there is torticollis, but rather placed simply in a position of comfort.

The use of multiple imaging modalities (conventional radiography, ultrasound, CT, and MR) is common in the radiologic workup of torticollis. Ultrasound is generally reserved for congenital torticollis, muscular issues, and to assess for potential infectious etiologies.

Plain radiography is the preferred initial imaging choice. The standard x-ray series consists of 3 views: AP, cross-table lateral, and open-mouth. The open mouth view is used to visualize C1, C2, and the atlantoaxial and atlanto-occipital articulations. This view is often difficult to obtain in young children, and proper positioning may prove difficult in any symptomatic patient with torticollis and restricted neck movement. If the patient can perform flexion and extension on his or her own without pain, these are the best views to assess for instability. In fact, outpatient screening for atlantoaxial subluxation in patients with Down syndrome consists of lateral neck radiographs taken in the neutral position and in flexion and extension. However, in the ED, forced flexion and extension should be avoided in symptomatic patients given the risk for acute subluxation. When evaluating x-rays, one should always assess the vertebral body height and alignment, the relationship of the lateral masses of the atlas and the dens, and centering of the dens in the open-mouth view, if obtained. If AARS or AARF is noted on x-ray, radiologists may use different degrees of classification based on the size of the shift.

A CT scan should be performed when the clinical suspicion of a cervical spine injury is high to assess for bony abnormalities. CT can be used to diagnose AARF by looking for facet displacement of the lateral atlantoaxial joints. Finally, MR is the modality of choice for assessing the supportive soft tissues of the spine and the spinal cord itself. It is also useful in evaluating for disruption of the alar and transverse ligaments. The best MR sequence is the fat saturation sequence to assess edema. Some institutions can also perform flexion and extension views during MRI. Any patient with neurologic symptoms should receive an emergent MR.

Screening for instability has been controversial and ever changing. More recent studies show that screening x-rays for instability have no predictive validity for future acute dislocation or subluxation at the atlantoaxial joint. In addition, some individuals that have radiologic atlantoaxial instability on one film have resolution on subsequent exams. Therefore, routine screening for asymptomatic patients with Trisomy 21 is no longer recommended, and asymptomatic patients should not be excluded from most sporting events. Nevertheless, most providers discourage activities that have high risk for cervical overflexion, such as diving and boxing, for children with Down syndrome.

Signs and symptoms with subluxation result from compression of nerve roots or the cord itself. Patients who present with symptoms of spinal cord compression may require immediate neurosurgery. Surgeons will decompress the spinal cord, reduce deformities, and perform internal fixation with fusion as indicated. Less severe instability is managed on a case-by-case basis, often with a rigid cervical collar and analgesia.

CASE CONCLUSION

Our patient was found to have ligamentous laxity causing an anterior subluxation of C1 on C2. MR confirmed this finding and showed a mass effect on the cord. He was taken to the OR for stabilization and did well postoperatively with resolution of his pain and neurologic symptoms.

KEY POINTS

- Children with Down syndrome generally have laxity of vertebral ligaments, potentially causing atlantoaxial instability, subluxation, and possibly, spinal cord compression.
- Any new neck pain, torticollis, decreased motor skills, or change in gait should prompt C-spine immobilization in the position of comfort and urgent imaging.

- X-rays should be performed with an attempt to obtain an open-mouth view if possible.
- CT will better assess the instability, and an MRI can assess the ligaments and spinal cord, if necessary.

Further Reading

1. Foley C, Killeen OG. Musculoskeletal anomalies. *Arch Dis Child*. 2019;104:482–487.
2. Cohen WI. Atlantoaxial instability, what's next? *Arch Pediatr Adolesc Med*. 1998;152:119.
3. Pueschel SM, Scola FH. Atlantoaxial instability in individuals with Down syndrome: epidemiologic, radiographic, and clinical studies. *Pediatrics*. 1987;80:555.
4. Cremers MJ, Bol E, de Roos F, van Gijn J. Risk of sports activities in children with Down's syndrome and atlantoaxial instability. *Lancet*. 1993;342(8870):511–514.
5. Pueschel SM, Scola FH, Pezzullo JC. A longitudinal study of atlanto-dens relationships in asymptomatic individuals with Down syndrome. *Pediatrics*. 1992;89(6 Pt 2):1194–1198.
6. Haque S, Bilal Shafi BB, Kaleem M. Imaging of torticollis in children. *Radiographics*. 2012;32(2):557–571.

*We would like to acknowledge Pediatric Neurosurgeon Dr. Shaun Rodgers for his appraisal of the text and up-to-date recommendations for spinal injuries.

17 Shouldn't This Be Connected?

Joshua Rocker and Anna Thomas

Case Study

A 5-year-old boy presents to the Emergency Department (ED) with facial injuries and altered mental status after being struck by a motor vehicle. He arrives at the trauma center in a cervical collar and is secured to a backboard receiving bag-valve-mask ventilation. The left chest has decreased breath sounds, so a chest tube is placed and 100mL of blood is collected. His initial heart rate is 110 BPM, blood pressure is 74/38mmHg, and he has palpable peripheral pulses. A brief neurological assessment demonstrates a minimally conscious (GCS of 5) child and therefore the airway is secured. Strength and sensation could not be assessed in the extremities prior to sedation and paralysis. Heart rate and blood pressure are grossly unchanged following chest tube placement and two 20mL/kg NS boluses and 1 10 mL/kg unit of packed red blood cells (PRBCs) are administered. An extended focused assessment with sonography for trauma (eFAST) exam does not reveal any fluid in the abdomen or any signs of pericardial effusion.

What do you do now?

DISCUSSION

Presenting to you is a young boy following a high-force trauma, found to have significant alteration in mental status requiring intubation for airway protection and signs of a pneumothorax requiring chest tube placement. Additionally, the patient is found to have significant hypotension, concerning for shock. Maintaining adequate perfusion is a critical part of the ABCs of trauma management. A provider must determine if the shock is hypovolemic from hemorrhage, obstructive from cardiac tamponade or tension pneumothorax, or neurogenic, most commonly due to a cervical spine injury. Hypovolemic shock and obstructive shock both typically present with hypotension and a compensatory tachycardia. Comparatively, our patient does not have tachycardia despite significant hypotension, and his vitals do not change despite attention to hypovolemia and hemorrhage with the two 20mL/kg NS boluses and 1 10 mL/kg unit of PRBCs. This makes obstructive or neurogenic shock higher on your differential. Obstructive shock may respond to fluid resuscitation, but response will depend on the degree of obstruction. An eFAST was performed, and there was no fluid seen in the abdomen; there was no sign of cardiac tamponade, and a chest tube was placed to reduce any tension pneumothorax; therefore, the persistent hypotension is most consistent with neurogenic shock. This type of shock is due to a loss of sympathetic signal from the spinal cord leading to vasodilation and hypotension, also known as distributive shock, much like what is seen in anaphylaxis. However, with no or limited sympathetic communication to increase the heart rate, these patients have hypotension and a lack of tachycardia that are often unresponsive to fluid resuscitation. This type of shock raises our already high concern for a cervical spine injury in this trauma patient.

The incidence of cervical spine injuries is much lower for children as compared to adults, 1% and 4%, respectively, but children have a much higher rate of serious sequelae from these injuries.[1,2] It has been reported that there is a 60% chance of pediatric C-spine injuries causing permanent neurologic damage and a 40%–50% chance of death.[2] Clinicians need to be vigilant and thoughtful regarding the evaluation and management of the pediatric patient with potential injury of the cervical spine.[3] The disproportionately large head sizes in younger children positions the fulcrum of cervical motion at C2–C3, leading to more upper-cervical spine injuries compared to children older than 8 years, where the fulcrum is lower at C5–C6. Also, younger children have relatively lax cervical ligaments, poorer muscle tone, and underdeveloped articular facets, increasing their predisposition for cervical spine instability with trauma. In our patient with a Glasgow Coma Scale (GCS) of 8 and the subsequent intubation with a sedative and a paralytic, a thorough neurological exam is near impossible. Although intracranial injuries are of the highest concern after blunt head trauma in patients with altered mental status, cervical spine stability must also be maintained, and neuroimaging of both the brain and C-spine are essential.

The Pediatric Emergency Care Applied Research Network (PECARN) identified 8 predictors associated with cervical spine injuries in pediatric patients following blunt trauma. Those predictors are: altered mental status, focal neurological deficit, neck pain, torticollis, substantial torso injury, predisposing medical conditions, diving injury mechanism, and high-risk motor vehicle collision as mechanism of injury.[4] Our patient meets 3 of these predictors portending C-spine injury: altered mental status, substantial torso injury, and mechanism of high-risk motor vehicle collision.

In addition to the radiographic evaluations our patient will receive of the head, chest, and abdomen/pelvis, our patient is unable to have his cervical spine clinically cleared while unresponsive, so his cervical spine is secured with a Miami-J collar, exchanging the one placed by EMS, and will require cervical spine imaging. There continues to be a lack of consensus on using plain films (lateral and anteroposterior (AP) +/– open-mouth, flexion, and extension views) or computed tomography (CT) scans for radiographic clearance of the cervical spine. However, for those with severe mechanisms of injury, polytrauma, or a GCS <8, as seen with our patient, several consensus statements agree that the initial choice of imaging would be a CT of the C-spine without contrast.[2,5,6] CT of the C-spine is very useful in this scenario to identify fractures and alignment, but also helps assess the craniocervical junction and soft tissues. In the trauma bay, our patient's hemodynamics improve after initiating phenylephrine for neurogenic shock refractory to fluid resuscitation, and he is then safely transported from the trauma bay to the CT scanner, where there are findings concerning for an atlanto-occipital distraction (AOD) injury.

Three key areas to closely evaluate on all C-spine CT examinations when evaluating a potential AOD injury are the atlanto-occipital interval, the basion-dental interval, and soft tissues of the cervical spine. The atlanto-occipital interval is the distance between the inferior cortical tip of the occipital condyle and the superior cortical margin of adjacent C1 facet which is measured on the sagittal plane images in bone windows. A normal atlanto-occipital interval on CT is <2.5mm and is best measured perpendicular to the atlanto-occipital joint space on sagittal imaging, being careful to avoid measurements at the level of the occipital condylar notch, which can artifactually elevate this value.[2] The atlanto-occipital interval is a sensitive and specific CT measurement for the detection of atlanto-occipital dissociation.[2,7,8] Next, the basion-dental interval, the distance between the inferior tip of the clivus/basion and the superior tip of the dens, is best measured on the midline sagittal plane CT image in bone windows. A normal basion-dental interval value on CT for children with an ossified os terminale is <9.5 mm and <11.6 mm in children without this ossification center.[7] The os terminale ossifies between 21 months and 10 years.[7] A widened basion-dental interval is highly suggestive of an AOD.[8] All physicians know the value of evaluating the bone window images for C-spine studies, but the value of the soft tissue windows is underappreciated. It is critical to look at the soft tissue windows for findings such as fluid elevating the tectorial membrane and stranding or edema in prevertebral, craniocervical, and paraspinal soft tissues, as these soft tissue signs may be indicative of a serious underlying cervical injury that is not able to be seen on CT.[2]

Imaging for this patient demonstrates classic findings of an AOD injury. First, the sagittal plane CT image in bone windows through the atlanto-occipital joint demonstrates a widened atlanto-occipital interval (Figure 17.1). Second, the midline sagittal plane CT image in bone windows shows a widened basion-dental interval of 32mm (Figure 17.2). Third, the sagittal CT image in soft tissue windows demonstrates an abnormally elevated tectorial membrane (arrow) which is bowed/lifted superiorly from its usual positioning due to mass effect from a retroclival epidural hemorrhage (Figure 17.3).

An AOD injury occurs when there is abnormal widening or distraction of the occiput from the atlas (C1). These injuries are typically seen in high-velocity motor vehicle collisions or when pedestrians are struck by vehicles.

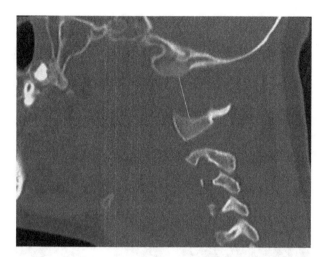

FIGURE 17.1. Sagittal plane CT image in bone windows through the atlanto-occipital joint demonstrates a widened atlanto-occipital interval (white line), the distance between the inferior cortical tip of the occipital condyle and the superior cortical margin of adjacent C1 facet (normal is less than 2.5mm).

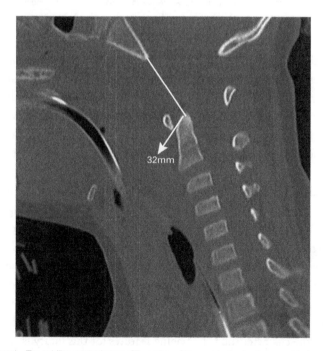

FIGURE 17.2. The midline sagittal plane CT section of the cervical spine in bone windows shows a widened basion-dental interval, the distance between the inferior tip of the clivus/basion and the superior tip of the dens measures 32mm (Normal is less than 9.5mm with ossified odontoid tip).

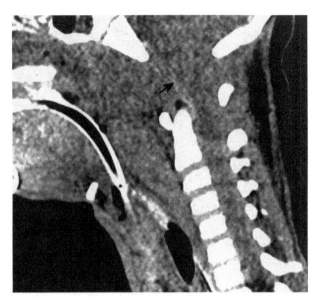

FIGURE 17.3. The midline sagittal plane CT section of the cervical spine in soft tissue window demonstrates an abnormally elevated tectorial membrane (arrow) which is bowed/lifted superiorly from its usual position due to retroclival epidural hemorrhage causing mass effect.

Due to the substantial forces involved and the proximity to the brainstem and potential for traumatic injury to the internal carotid arteries and vertebral arteries, these injuries are often associated with a high mortality prior to arrival to the ED for medical care. In those patients that do present to an ED, AOD is rarely an isolated finding, with other severe traumatic brain, spinal, vascular, or solid organ injuries also contributing to high in-hospital morbidity and mortality.

Providers must have a high index of suspicion for these injuries in young children who have sustained high-energy traumas, as there is a significant risk for devastating neurological damage if unrecognized and because the neurological exam can vary widely, from paraplegia to asymptomatic.[9] CT of the cervical spine is often the first study performed to assess cervical spine integrity in these patients in the emergent setting. However, classic signs of cervical spine fractures or malalignment on CT, which many physicians are adept at identifying, may be absent in patients with AOD. As such, understanding the characteristic CT imaging features for this injury is critical.

As atlanto-occipital injuries are primarily ligamentous injuries, which are seen better on MR imaging, further imaging is often performed with non-contrast MRI. This is done to either confirm the diagnosis in cases when CT imaging is not definitive and clinical concerns remain, or to further evaluate the ligamentous structures which primarily maintain the stability of the atlanto-occipital junction. Subsequent imaging by MRI is especially important for obtunded or sedated patients in whom a neurological exam cannot be performed. Despite a negative CT, the laxity of the cervical spine in young children may allow for a spinal cord injury without radiographic abnormalities (SCIWORA), which may not be appreciated in these patients with blunted neurological exams.

Management of a patient with an AOD injury will depend on the available resources of the treating facility and the concomitant injuries the patient sustained. Clinical stabilization and potential transfer to a hospital with pediatric neurosurgical, critical care, or other subspecialty services may be required. Proper fitting cervical collars, often a challenge for young children, are even more critical in the management of AOD injuries, as the collar itself has the potential to worsen the distraction of the occiput.[10]

Further management outside the ED typically involves cervical immobilization by halo or cervicothoracic orthosis, and if instability is suspected, spinal fusion may be required. Unfortunately, outcomes data are limited, but children appear to have better survival and neurological outcomes than adults.[11] Additionally, presenting features appear to offer some prediction of outcomes in those who survive to discharge. Two reviews found that children presenting with neurological deficits or MRI findings of spinal cord injuries generally had marginal long-term improvements. Conversely, those presenting with no neurological deficits or only signs of traumatic brain injury generally had no long-term deficits at follow-up.[11,12]

For this patient, he was initially resuscitated in the ED and transferred to the pediatric intensive care unit, where a halo stabilization device was placed by pediatric neurosurgery at the bedside. Unfortunately, the patient succumbed to his injuries and died on hospital day 2.

- Neurogenic shock should be suspected in the trauma patient with persistent hypotension, lack of tachycardia, and lack of responsiveness to treating hypovolemic or hemorrhagic shock.
- Pediatric cervical spine injuries following blunt trauma, though rare, have a high risk for devastating neurological sequelae.
- The 8 factors predicting a possible pediatric c-spine injuries in those who suffer blunt trauma are: altered mental status, focal neurological deficit, neck pain, torticollis, substantial torso injury, predisposing medical conditions, diving injury mechanism, and high-risk motor vehicle collision as mechanism of injury.

- The initial evaluation of cervical spine injury should be performed with a non-contrast c-spine CT with particular attention given to atlanto-occipital interval, basion-dental interval, and soft tissues, as these are key indicators for underlying atlanto-occipital distraction injuries.
- In a sedated or unconscious patient it is important to maintain C-spine immobilization, even following a normal or negative CT scan. An MRI is necessary to rule out ligamentous instability or SCIWORA.

References

1. Leonard JR, Jaffe DM, Kuppermann N, et al.; Pediatric Emergency Care Applied Research Network (PECARN) Cervical Spine Study Group. Cervical spine injury patterns in children. *Pediatrics*. 2014;133(5):e1179–e1188.
2. McAllister AS, Nagaraj U, Rhadhakrishnan R. Emergent imaging of pediatric cervical spine trauma. *Radiographics*. 2019;29:1126–1142.
3. Nitecki S, Moir CR. Predictive factors of the outcome of traumatic cervical spine fracture in children. *J Pediatr Surg*. 1994;29:1409–1411.
4. Leonard JC, Kuppermann N, Olsen C, et al.; Pediatric Emergency Care Applied Research Network. Factors associated with cervical spine injury in children after blunt trauma. *Ann Emerg Med*. 2011;58(2):145–155.

5. Chung S, Mikrogianakis A, Wales PW, et al. Trauma Association of Canada Pediatric Subcommittee National Pediatric Cervical Spine Evaluation Pathway: Consensus guidelines. *J Trauma*. 2011;70(4):873–884.

6. Herman MJ, Brown KO, Sponseller PD, et al. Pediatric cervical spine clearance: a consensus statement and algorithm from the Pediatric Cervical Spine Clearance Working Group. *J Bone Joint Surg*. 2019;101(1):e1.

7. Bertozzi JC, Rojas CA, Martinez CR. Evaluation of the pediatric craniocervical junction on MDCT. *Am J Roentgenol*. 2009;192:26–31.

8. Riascos R, Bonfante E, Cotes C, et al. Imaging of atlanto-occipital and atlantoaxial traumatic injuries: what the radiologist needs to know. *Radiographics*. 2015;35:2121–2134.

9. Filiberto DM, Sharpe JP, Croce MA, et al. Traumatic atlanto-occipital dissociation: no longer a death sentence. *Surgery*. 2018;164:500–503.

10. Dickman CA, Papadopoulos SM, Sonntag VKH, et al. Traumatic Occipitoatlantal Dislocations. *J Spinal Disord*. 1993;6(4):300–313.

11. Horn EM, Feiz-Efan I, Lekovic GP, et al. Survivors of occipitoatlantal dislocation injuries: imaging and clinical correlates. *J Neurosurg: Spine*. 2007;6:113–120.

12. Sun PP, Poffenbarger GJ, Durham S, et al. Spectrum of occipitoatlantoaxial injury in young children. *J Neurosurg*. 2000;93(1 Suppl):28–39.

18 Head First into the Pool

Aaron McAllister and Kristol Das

Case Study

A 15-year-old girl with a history of depression was reported missing by her family. She was found naked in cold water under an 80-foot-tall bridge by a passerby 1 hour after being reported missing. It was a presumed suicide attempt, with her clothes found on the bridge. The jump/fall was unwitnessed, and it is unknown whether she lost consciousness. She presents to your facility as a level 1 trauma. Primary survey is notable for mildly diminished breath sounds at bilateral bases and a capillary refill of 3 seconds distally. Her Glasgow Coma Scale (GCS) is 15. The secondary survey is notable for tenderness to palpation at the base of the cervical spine and along the thoracic spine. She also has diffuse tenderness to her abdomen and noted 4/5 strength to bilateral upper extremities with elbow flexion and extension. She has 3/5 shoulder abduction on the right. In addition, she describes shortness of breath and intermittent numbness and paresthesia to her extremities, along with right ankle, back, and neck pain.

What do you do now?

DISCUSSION

Given the condition in which the patient was found and the fall/jump from height, a complete trauma evaluation is indicated. Management and evaluation priorities, as with any other trauma patient, are stabilization of life threats before moving on to address other injuries. This patient was placed in an appropriately sized cervical collar at the conclusion of the primary survey. She remained hemodynamically stable with a negative FAST examination and normal complete blood count (CBC), liver function tests (LFTs), and lipase. Due to the height of the fall and clinical findings, computed tomography (CT) scans of chest, abdomen, pelvis, and spine were obtained. Here, we will focus on the evaluation and management of her spinal injuries.

In the acute stabilization period, if there is suspicion for a cervical spine injury, a pediatric trauma patient should be positioned supine with a rigid collar and lateral immobilization. While the National Emergency X-radiography Use Study (NEXUS) and Canadian C-spine (CCR) rules are often applied, there is no validated decision tool for pediatric cervical spine clearance (Table 18.1). These decision rules are not universally applicable to children due to anatomic and physiologic differences between children and adults. Skeletally immature patients have a less rigid spine, injuries are more likely to be soft tissue and ligamentous, and they are at increased risk of spinal cord injury without radiographic abnormality (SCIWORA). In addition, the level of spinal injury is typically higher in children as the fulcrum of the cervical spine is higher. It is approximately at C2–C3 in infants and moves to C5–C6 typically by age 8, as found in adults.

The Pediatric Emergency Care Applied Research Network (PECARN) retrospectively identified 8 factors associated with cervical spine injury in children 0–16 years old, as shown in Table 18.1. Utilizing these data and decision tools, further evaluation of our patient is indicated given her neurologic deficit, neck pain, and mechanism of injury. Moreover, in a prospective analysis, the PECARN group found that diving, axial load, neck pain, inability to move neck, intubation, or respiratory distress were 92% sensitive and 50.3% specific for cervical spinal injury. Alternatively, absent pain, neurologic deficit, or radiographic abnormalities, the cervical collar can be removed.

TABLE 18.1   **Decision tools for cervical spine clearance**

NEXUS (high-risk criteria)	CCR*** (high-risk criteria)	PECARN**** risk factors
Focal deficits	GCS <15	Altered mental status
Midline tenderness	Age >65	Focal neurologic deficits
Altered mental status	Fall >3 feet	Neck pain
Intoxication	Axial load to the head	Torticollis
Distracting injuries**	High speed MVC	Substantial torso injury
	Paresthesia	Predisposing condition
	Neck pain/tenderness	for C-spine injury
		High-risk MVC
		Diving

** long bone fracture, visceral injury, large laceration, crush injury, burns
*** Canadian Cervical Spine Rule
**** Pediatric Emergency Care Applied Research Network
MVC = motor vehicle collision.

X-ray is the initial imaging modality of choice in children under 16 years of age. Standard views are the anteroposterior (AP), lateral, and open-mouth views. The lateral view is the most sensitive and specific and can be used as an initial screening image, with additional views obtained if it reveals suspicious findings or the patient has persistent pain. The open-mouth odontoid view can be difficult to obtain and has limited diagnostic utility in children younger than 5 years old, making AP and lateral views sufficient in this age cohort. Patients with an identified single-level injury should have radiography with at least 4 levels above and below the level of the fracture.

In children with radiographic abnormalities on x-ray, persistent pain in the setting of polytrauma, high-risk mechanism, or altered mental status, CT imaging is indicated. Due to our patient's mechanism of injury and concerning findings on secondary survey, CT imaging of her chest, abdomen, and pelvis were indicated. Note that CT imaging of the spine minimally contributes to radiation dose in patients who get concurrent CT imaging of the trunk, as the spine images are extracted from the same imaged volume. The incremental radiation dose is only for the portions of the spine not included in the trunk-imaged volume. Despite its sensitivity for bony injury, the pediatric cervical spine cannot be cleared with CT alone in the setting of high-risk trauma, as CT is not as sensitive for soft-tissue injuries.

Due to the mechanism of injury in our patient (fall from height), CT was the first dedicated imaging of the spine, performed in conjunction with CT of the chest, abdomen, and pelvis. The chest, abdomen, and pelvis showed bilateral pneumothoraces and a grade I splenic injury. CT of the spine demonstrated a fracture of the right C1 lamina, burst fracture of C7 with retropulsion of osseous fragments, resulting in spinal canal narrowing, and compression fractures of T1, T2, and L2 (Figures 18.1–18.4). These spinal fractures are all consistent with an axial loading injury (vertical compression mechanism). Additional clinical history revealed the patient believes she had an oblique headfirst water entry with first impact on the right occiput.

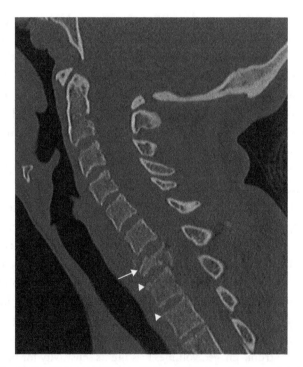

FIGURE 18.1. Sagittal CT demonstrating burst fracture at C7 (arrow) with associated spinal canal narrowing. Also note compression fractures of T1 and T2 (arrowheads).

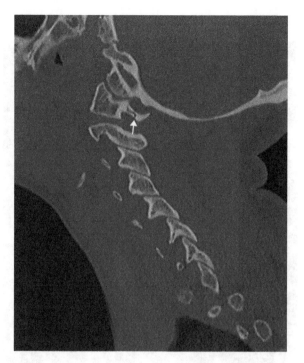

FIGURE 18.2. Sagittal CT image of unilateral C1 lamina fracture (arrow).

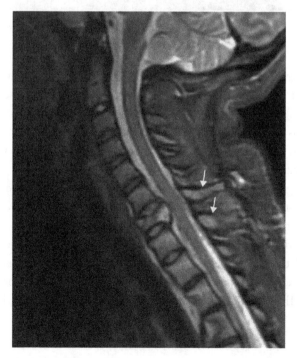

FIGURE 18.3. Sagittal MRI STIR sequence demonstrating burst fracture of C7, compression fractures of T1, T2, and T3 with associated edema in the spinous processes (arrows).

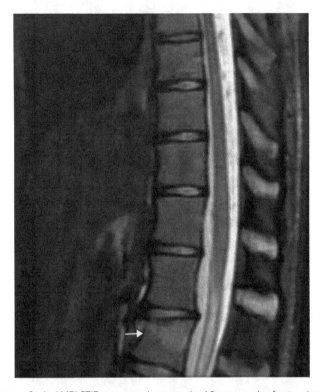

FIGURE 18.4. Sagittal MRI STIR sequence demonstrating L2 compression fracture (arrow).

Angiography should be added in high-energy mechanisms that may cause sudden or prolonged neck hyperextension or rotation, as these may also precipitate vertebral artery injury such as dissection or pseudoaneurysm. Symptoms of vertebral artery dissection include neck pain, occipital headaches, and neurologic deficits that may be delayed up to 1 week from the trauma.

CT angiography of the head and neck was performed in our patient secondary to the axial loading mechanism of injury and multiple identified spinal fractures. No vascular injuries were identified.

Magnetic resonance imaging (MRI) is the modality of choice for evaluation of the soft tissues, spinal cord, intervertebral discs, bone marrow, and ligaments, and can differentiate between spinal cord hemorrhage and edema. MRI is indicated in the setting of neurologic deficits, in injuries associated with cord injury or ligamentous injury, such as burst fractures for better delineating CT or plain film findings, preoperative planning, or to further evaluate clinical findings not explained by previous imaging. Direct visualization of the osseous cortex by MRI is inferior to CT. Fractures on MRI are identified by osseous deformation or secondary findings such as marrow edema or adjacent soft tissue edema. For direct osseous visualization, CT is preferred; however, secondary findings such as marrow edema may be the only finding in subtle fractures. Moreover, MRI can better visualize the bone components that have not yet ossified, such as the physes or apophyses. The primary limitations of MRI are long scan times and the need for sedation in patients who cannot lie still for the requisite scan time due to age or medical condition.

In addition to weakness on neurologic exam, our patient had a unilateral C1 fracture and multiple compression fractures, including a burst fracture of C7 with retropulsed bone fragments, the presumed cause of the neurological deficits on presentation. An urgent MRI of the spine was performed.

MRI demonstrated the burst fracture of C7. The spinal cord was displaced posteriorly by the retropulsed bone fragment but was normal in signal. Edema noted in the C6–C7 interspinous space and within the posterior longitudinal ligament was concerning for ligamentous sprain. Marrow edema was noted in the vertebra at T1, T2, T3, and L2, consistent with compression fractures identified on CT. The C1 lamina fracture was not as well delineated by MRI as on CT. The MRI also showed edema at the C6 vertebral body suspicious for an additional compression fracture not visible by CT. An apophyseal avulsion fracture of the spinous process of C7 was also identified, not visible by CT. The pattern of spinal injuries observed was again compatible with an axial loading mechanism of injury.

Axial loading injuries occur when a compressive force is applied along the long axis of the patient. Diving injuries are a quintessential example, but other mechanisms include fall from a height, motor vehicle collision (MVC; i.e., impact of head on roof of car), or a heavy object falling on the head. Axial loading can occur with both head-first or feet-first impacts; however, injuries in head-first impacts are more severe. In the case of diving, axial loading occurs with abrupt deceleration of the head and continued forward momentum of the torso and limbs exerting compression forces along the long axis of the body. Jefferson fractures, the eponym given to burst fractures of C1 (rare in children), are the classically reported injury of axial loading. Our case is unusual in that the C1 fracture is unilateral; usually the C1 ring breaks in 2 or more places. Vertebral compression fractures are perhaps the most common axial loading injury and involve multiple vertebrae 20% of the time. Moreover, clinical assessment only has a sensitivity of 81% and specificity of 68% in children. Thus, if one compression fracture is identified on imaging in a clinically significant trauma, consider imaging the remainder of the spine. Twisting, flexion, or extension at the time of impact can affect the fracture pattern. Severe compression fractures that involve the posterior vertebral body cortex are burst fractures. Retropulsion of bone fragments of a burst fracture into the spinal canal can cause spinal cord injury/compression, potentially leading to neurological deficits.

Our patient was stabilized and monitored with mean arterial pressure (MAP) maintained >75mmHg until the following morning, when the patient was taken to the operating room for C7 corpectomy with C6–T1 anterior instrumentation and fusion.

KEY POINTS

· Skeletally immature patients have a less rigid spine and increased risk of soft tissue and ligamentous injury rather than osseous injuries.

TIPS FROM THE RADIOLOGIST

· AP/lateral x-rays of the cervical spine are the initial imaging study of choice in children with suspected cervical spine injury.
· Negative CT imaging does not clear the pediatric cervical spine if high clinical suspicion for injury remains.
· MRI is indicated in the setting of neurologic deficits, in injuries associated with cord injury or ligamentous injury, for better delineating CT or plain film findings, preoperative planning, or to further evaluate clinical findings not explained by previous imaging.

Further Reading

1. Nadja Kadom, Susan Palasis, Sumit Pruthi, et al. Suspected spine trauma-child. Available at https://acsearch.acr.org/docs/3101274/Narrative/. American College of Radiology. Accessed April 26, 2021.

2. Gary R. Fleisher, Stephen Ludwig, eds. *Textbook of Pediatric Emergency Medicine*. 6th ed. (Philadelphia: Lippincott Williams & Wilkins; 2010). Available from: Books@Ovid at http://ovidsp.ovid.com. Accessed April 26, 2021.

3. Expert Panel on Neurological Imaging and Musculoskeletal Imaging: Beckmann NM, West OC, et al. ACR Appropriateness Criteria® suspected spine trauma. *J Am Coll Radiol*. 2019;16(5S):S264–S285. doi: 10.1016/j.jacr.2019.02.002.

4. Fleisher GR, Ludwig S, eds. *Textbook of Pediatric Emergency Medicine*. 6th ed. Philadelphia: Lippincott Williams & Wilkins; 2010.

5. Hoffman JR, Mower WR, Wolfson AB, Todd KH, Zucker MI. Validity of a set of clinical criteria to rule out injury to the cervical spine in patients with blunt trauma. National Emergency X-Radiography Utilization Study Group [published correction appears in *N Engl J Med*. 2001 Feb 8;344(6):464]. *N Engl J Med*. 2000;343(2):94–99. doi: 10.1056/NEJM200007133430203.

6. Leonard JC, Browne LR, Ahmad FA, et al. Cervical spine injury risk factors in children with blunt trauma. *Pediatrics*. 2019;144(1). doi: 10.1542/peds.2018-3221, 10.1542/peds.2018-3221

7. McAllister AS, Nagaraj U, Radhakrishnan R. Emergent imaging of pediatric cervical spine trauma. *Radiographics*. 2019;39(4):1126–1142. doi: 10.1148/rg.2019180100.

8. Stiell IG, Clement CM, McKnight RD, et al. The Canadian C-spine rule versus the NEXUS low-risk criteria in patients with trauma. *N Engl J Med*. 2003;349(26):2510–2518. doi: 10.1056/NEJMoa031375.

19 Pain in the Back

Deanna Margius, Sophia Gorgens, David Foster, and Shankar Srinivas Ganapathy

Case Study

A 10-year-old previously healthy boy, JT, presents to you with low back pain. He enjoys sports and plays football in the fall, wrestling in the winter, and lacrosse in the spring. Over the past 3 months, JT has noticed an intermittent nagging lower back pain, present most days. He presents to the Emergency Department (ED) today because the pain has been persistent for the past 3 days and woke him up last night. JT was born full-term with no complications, is up to date on vaccinations, and has never been hospitalized. Physical exam is notable for tenderness to palpation at L5, mild lumbar scoliosis, a normal neurological exam, and normal vital signs.

What do I do now?

DIFFERENTIAL DIAGNOSIS FOR PEDIATRIC BACK PAIN

The most common causes of pediatric back pain include musculoskeletal conditions and trauma. However, there are more worrisome etiologies that cannot be missed. It is crucial to assess for red flags by history and physical exam (Box 19.1).[1] In general, imaging is deemed unnecessary when there are no red flags present, the back pain is acute, there is no associated trauma, and the child's physical exam, including a full neurological exam, is normal.[1] On the other hand, imaging is necessary when there are red flags present (see Box 19.1), the back pain is persistent, there is associated trauma, or the child's physical exam or lab workup shows abnormalities.[1]

When approaching a child with back pain, remember to keep a broad differential. Although spondylolysis and spondylolisthesis are the most common diagnosable causes of low back pain in children, other causes to consider include: trauma resulting in vertebral fractures, dislocations, or ligamentous injuries; intervertebral disc herniation; Scheuermann disease (osteochondrosis); inflammatory disorders such as acute transverse myelitis; discitis or osteomyelitis from infectious etiologies, most often bacterial; and benign or malignant neoplasm such as leukemias or neuroblastoma.[1] Many of these pathologies can also be associated with spondylolisthesis, but they will usually present in the setting of additional signs and symptoms.

In the case of JT, concerning findings include pain severe enough to wake him up at night, pain that has been persistent for 3 months, and point tenderness at L5. All these factors warrant imaging, as the differential diagnosis for JT is currently broad and includes spondylolysis/spondylolisthesis,

---

BOX 19.1 **Red Flags in the History-Taking of a Child with Back Pain**

Back Pain Red Flags
Duration >4 weeks
Fevers, chills, night sweats
Pain worse at night
Point tenderness
Neuro exam focal deficits
Cancer history
Radiation history

---

vertebral body fracture, or neoplasm, with infectious etiologies lower on the differential due to a lack of systemic symptoms such as fevers or chills.

SPONDYLOLYSIS AND SPONDYLOLISTHESIS: DEFINITION

Spondylolysis is a weakness or fracture in the pars interarticularis of the vertebral arch.[2] If left untreated, this condition can progress to spondylolisthesis, where the vertebral body becomes displaced anteriorly.[2] This occurs more frequently when there are bilateral pars interarticularis fractures.[2] Although spondylolysis can occur at any vertebrae, the most commonly affected are L5 and L4.[2] Spondylolysis and spondylolisthesis are grouped into categories based on mechanism by the Wiltse classification (Table 19.1).[3]

Furthermore, spondylolysis and spondylolisthesis can be further classified by amount of vertebral displacement through the Meyerding grading system (Table 19.2).[4] The edge of the vertebra inferior to the displaced vertebra is divided into 4 quarters, corresponding to 25%, 50%, 75%, and 100% dislocation.[4] The posteroinferior corner of the dislocated vertebra will become displaced anteriorly, along the edge of the inferior vertebra.[4] When referring to the type and grade of the disease, the grade is stated, along with the formal name of the mechanism.[4]

TABLE 19.1 **Wiltse Classification for Types of Spondylolysis/ Spondylolisthesis and Their Mechanisms**

Type	Name of Mechanism	Description
Type 1	Congenital dysplasia	Congenital attenuation of pars interarticularis
Type 2	Isthmic	Stress fractures and repetitive fractures of pars interarticularis
Type 3	Degenerative	Degeneration of intervertebral discs leads to chronic instability
Type 4	Traumatic	Fracture in region other than pars interarticularis
Type 5	Pathologic (tumors or osteoporosis)	Disease process that disrupts the spinal structure, malignancy, infectious, or immunological condition

TABLE 19.2 **Meyerding Grading System for Spondylolisthesis**

Grade	Percent Translation of Cranial Vertebra
I	0%–25%
II	25%–50%
III	50%–75%
IV	75%–100%

EPIDEMIOLOGY AND RISK FACTORS

Spondylolysis and spondylolisthesis occur in approximately 6% of the population, including children and adults, and constitute 50% of low back pain diagnoses in preadolescent and adolescent athletes.[2] The cause is multifactorial, with a mix of genetic and environmental factors.[5] The Wiltse classification (Table 19.1) determines multiple different causes for this condition. Spondylolysis and spondylolisthesis occur more commonly in male athletes, as well as those who participate in activities that involve repeated hyperextension; these sports include dancing, diving, football, gymnastics, weightlifting, and wrestling. Repeated stress on the lumbar spine is more likely to cause strain on the pars interarticularis, leading to uni- or bilateral fractures. Additionally, kyphosis maintains posture in extension and is another risk factor for this disease.[6] It is believed that there is some genetic component, based on multiple cases occurring within the same family. Additionally, there is a higher prevalence of disease in the Eskimo population (50%), with a larger proportion of this group requiring surgical intervention.[5] The role of genetics in this disease process is a topic for future research, as specific genes have yet to be identified.

CLINICAL PRESENTATION

Most cases present asymptomatically and are identified as an incidental finding. Symptomatic patients typically present with midline low back pain that is exacerbated by physical activity, especially hyperextension movements. There is no relation between severity of pain and amount of vertebral dislocation. An additional clinical tool is the Stork Test, where the patient stands on one leg and extends the back. The test is positive if this maneuver elicits low back pain.[2] Additional clinical findings, although rare, include radicular pain, neurogenic claudication, and altered posture. The Phalen-Dickson signal occurs when the patient bends at the knees and hips. This posturing is due to the shortening of hamstrings, verticalization of the sacrum, and increased lordosis.[6]

DIAGNOSTIC WORKUP

When ordering imaging in children, radiation exposure is important to consider. Effective radiation dose—that is, the amount of radiation absorbed by the body—is measured in Sieverts (Sv). Although computed tomography (CT) is the gold standard for assessing the spine, a CT scan of the lumbar spine results in an effective dose of 19.15 mSv, while plain films collectively only result in approximately 3.7 mSv (2.20 mSv for an anterioposterior [AP] film and 1.50 mSv for a lateral film).[1,8] Therefore, first-line imaging in children with back pain should be plain films. Magnetic resonance imaging (MRI), which has no associated radiation, is expensive and time-consuming but may be considered as the follow-up study to an x-ray or if the x-ray studies are inconclusive or negative.[9,10] Additionally, remember that the choice of imaging modality depends on the differential diagnosis. If there is high clinical suspicion for spinal cord injury given the presence of neurological abnormalities, MRI is the test of choice rather than plain films.

As mentioned, imaging should be ordered when red flag symptoms are present. The first test ordered is typically a 2-view of the lumbar spine, AP and lateral (Figures 19.1a and 19.1b). Additional oblique views nearly double the radiation dose. Spondylolysis or spondylolisthesis, if present, is usually seen in the AP and lateral views. However, in patients with high BMI or recurrent back pain that have negative initial 2-view radiographs, oblique views may be of additional benefit in depicting the pars defects.[10] Radiologists assess for two findings: fracture or defect in the pars interarticularis and the presence of vertebral displacement. In the oblique

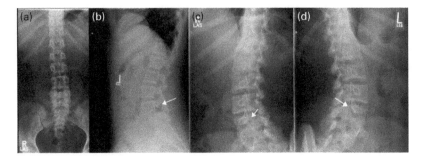

FIGURES 19.1a, 19.1b, 19.1c, 19.1d. AP (a) and lateral (b) views and bilateral oblique x-rays (c, d) views of lumbar spine show bilateral L5 spondylolysis (arrows) with Grade 1–2 spondylolisthesis of L5 over S1.

view, the pars interarticularis is analyzed. The "Scottie dog sign" describes a normal appearance of the vertebra in oblique projection. The pars interarticularis, which represents the neck of the dog, will have a lucency, signifying a fracture or defect in patients with spondylolysis (Figures 19.1c and 19.1d). This appears as a line through the neck of the dog.[2]

Additional advanced imaging may include bone scintigraphy with single-photon emission computed tomography (SPECT) or SPECT/CT, and MRI. MRI offers the advantage of depicting marrow edema, which helps assess if the pars fracture is acute or not, but it is rarely performed in an emergency setting or as an initial exam in a child with back pain unless there are acute neurologic signs or symptoms.[2] Bone scintigraphy with SPECT or SPECT/CT is an alternative to MRI which shows increased radiotracer uptake in the setting of acute pars fracture and other pathologies that can cause back pain, but it has a higher radiation dose than x-rays and should not be ordered as the initial study.[2] All of these modalities are more sensitive than radiographs and are therefore recommended only if radiographs do not identify fracture or displacement in the setting of high pretest probability for disease. It is not unusual for radiographs to yield false negative results, particularly with stress fractures or minimally displaced fractures.[2] Early imaging provides a baseline for disease type and grading, which can be useful for analyzing disease progression over time.[2] Keep in mind that the majority of mechanical low back pain in the pediatric population, especially in adolescents, is not associated with a radiologically diagnosable pathology.[9] Be judicious in who you refer for further imaging if initial x-rays are negative.

In the case of JT, as seen in Figures 19.1a, 19.1b, 19.1c, and 19.1d, x-rays were done in the ED and revealed bilateral L5 spondylolysis with Grade 1–2 spondylolisthesis of L5 over S1, where S1 was the transitional vertebra. This clinched the diagnosis for spondylolysis/spondylolisthesis, and JT did not require further imaging. A CT at this point would have exposed the patient to unnecessary additional radiation. JT was given pain control in the ED and was referred appropriately to orthopedics for outpatient management.

TREATMENT

Multiple factors impact disease management, including clinical symptoms, and both the presence and grade of vertebral displacement. Generally, spondylolysis alone does not require surgical management; treatment is usually conservative.[7] The first steps include pain control and physical therapy, with activity restrictions and bracing as needed.[7] Healing of fractured pars interarticularis fractures may be accelerated by interventions which increase blood flow to the spine; these include pulsed ultrasound and electrical bone stimulators.[2] Rehabilitation exercises that strengthen muscles in the abdomen and thighs may also improve pain.[6] Outpatient office visits should assess for clinical improvement and re-image the spine only if symptoms are worsening or not improving.[9] Plain films remain first line for follow-up imaging.[10]

Conservative management is not always effective for fractures that are wide, fragmented, or sclerotic, or spondylolisthesis with high grade displacement. In these cases, patients may need surgical correction with direct repair of the pars interarticularis or fusion of mobile segments of the spinal column.[3] Additional indications for surgery include unrelenting pain, progressive dislocation of the vertebra, neurological abnormalities, and spinal instability.[2] The long-term outlook for patients with spondylolysis/spondylolisthesis is usually favorable.[3, 9] A multidisciplinary team is involved in care, including pediatricians, rehabilitation specialists, and possibly spine surgeons in cases of failed conservative management.

Thankfully, in JT's case, the patient responded well to conservative management, receiving both adequate pain control and physical therapy for several weeks with consistent outpatient follow-up appointments with his orthopedist. His symptoms improved without the need for surgical intervention—or a repeat ED visit.

KEY POINTS

- Children with low back pain require a thorough history and physical examination to assess for red flag signs and symptoms.
- Spondylolysis and spondylolisthesis are the most common cause of low back pain in children, constituting 50% of all diagnoses in pre-adolescent and adolescent athletes.
- Treatment for both spondylolysis and spondylolisthesis depends on severity, but regardless, long-term outlook is usually favorable.

TIPS FOR THE RADIOLOGIST

- First-line imaging is by AP and lateral plain radiographs of the lumbar spine, with additional oblique views in selected cases.
- Lateral views should be reviewed for pars interarticularis defects and spondylolisthesis.
- Pars defects manifest as lucency through the pars (aka neck of Scottie dog) on oblique views.
- Reserve MRI and SPECT/CT for highly suspicious cases with negative radiographs, in the setting of high pretest probability.

References
1. Calloni SF, et al. Back pain and scoliosis in children: When to image, what to consider. *Neuroradiol J.* 2017;30(5):393–404. doi: 10.1177/1971400917697503.
2. Syrmou E, et al. Spondylolysis: a review and reappraisal. *Hippokratia.* 2010;14(1):17–21.
3. Wiltse LL. Classification, Terminology and measurements in spondylolisthesis. *Iowa Orthop J.* 1981;1:52–57. PMCID: PMC2328707.

‌

4. Meyerding HW. Spondylolisthesis. *Surg Gynecol Obstet*. 1932;54:371–377.

5. Tower S, et al. Spondylolysis and associated spondylolisthesis in Eskimo and Athabascan populations. *Clin Orthop Relat Res*. 1990;250:171–175.

6. Tebet MA. Current concepts on the sagittal balance and classification of spondylolysis and spondylolisthesis. *Rev Bras Ortop*. 2014 Feb 18;49(1):3–12. doi: 10.1016/j.rboe.2014.02.003.

7. Gagnet P, et al. Spondylolysis and spondylolisthesis: A review of the literature. *J Orthop*. 2018 Mar 17;15(2):404–407. doi: 10.1016/j.jor.2018.03.008

8. Scott MC, et al. Radiation exposure with spine imaging. *Contemp Spine Surg*. 2019 Nov;20(11): 1–7. doi: 10.1097/01.CSS.0000604020.74681.7a.

9. Miller R, et al. Imaging modalities for low back pain in children: a review of spondyloysis and undiagnosed mechanical back pain. *J Pediatr Orthop*. 2013 Apr–May;33(3):282–288. doi: 10.1097/BPO.0b013e318287fffb. PMID: 23482264.

10. Tofte JN, et al. Imaging pediatric spondylolysis: a systematic review. *Spine (Phila Pa 1976)*. 2017 May 15;42(10):777–782. doi: 10.1097/BRS.0000000000001912. PMID: 27669047.

20 Why Is This Infant So Fussy?

Michelle Greene, Anna Thomas, and Berkeley Bennett

Case Study

A 2-month-old female presents to the Emergency Department (ED) with vomiting and fussiness. Her birth was a full-term spontaneous vaginal delivery without complications. She passed meconium within 24 hours of birth. She drinks 2 ounces every few hours and has no history of spitting up. Mother states the vomiting started 48 hours ago, is nonbloody, nonbilious, and progressing in frequency. Today the baby is fussy and refusing oral intake. Her last stool was today and nonbloody. Mother reports a red spot in one eye 3 weeks ago that was not present at birth. The mother denies any previous trauma. Review of systems is negative for: fever, upper respiratory symptoms, cough, constipation, and diarrhea. On physical examination, the baby is irritable, especially with position changes, but consolable. There is a tear of the upper labial frenulum, which the mother reports was caused by the baby scratching herself. The rest of the exam is normal, including vital signs. There is no abdominal distension or tenderness.

What do you do now?

INTRODUCTION

The differential diagnosis for a vomiting infant is vast. A common benign cause is physiologic gastroesophageal reflux disease, otherwise known as a "happy spitter." The rapid progression of our patient's vomiting, associated irritability, and refusing oral intake suggest another, more serious condition. Hypertrophic pyloric stenosis presents with frequent emesis but is more common in male infants who usually retain their desire to eat and present with progressive vomiting that becomes increasingly forceful (projectile). Hirschsprung's disease can present with vomiting, but the history of passing meconium in the first 24 hours and no history of subsequent constipation makes this less likely. Adrenal insufficiency can also cause vomiting in an infant, but usually presents within the first 4 weeks of life. Food-protein in-duced enteropathy can cause vomiting, but typically presents with bloody stools. Intestinal obstruction is another life-threatening cause of vomiting in an infant and may be present even without bilious emesis. Intracranial pathology such as hydrocephalus or intracranial hemorrhage (ICH) can also cause emesis.

What do you do now?

Consider an acute abdominal series. Abdominal radiographs can pro-vide a quick assessment of the bowel gas pattern, so you obtain an acute abdominal series, which includes a chest x-ray. The abdominal x-rays (not shown) reveal a nonobstructive bowel gas pattern with air seen throughout nondilated small and large bowel loops. The chest x-ray demonstrates mul-tiple acute and healing rib fractures (Figure 20.1).

What do you do now?

A non-contrast head computed tomography (CT) scan is indicated. Intracranial pathology can be a cause of vomiting in infants, and the finding of acute and healing rib fractures without a trauma history raises concern for abusive head injury. A non-contrast head CT (Figures 20.2 and 20.3) is obtained.

CLASSIFICATION AND PATHOPHYSIOLOGY OF EXTRA-AXIAL HEMORRHAGE

The three most common types of post-traumatic extra-axial collec-tions are subdural, epidural, and subarachnoid collections. There are

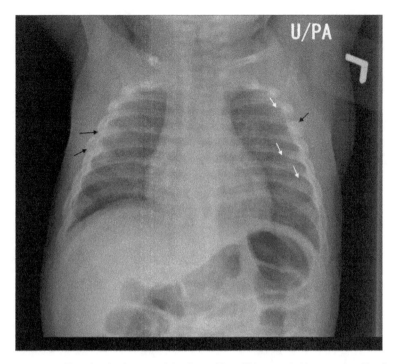

FIGURE 20.1. Frontal projection x-ray of the chest with multiple acute (white arrows) and healing (black arrows) rib fractures.

characteristic imaging features (described below) which help differentiate these three collections. Of the three different types of extra-axial collections, subdural collections are most encountered in the setting of abusive head trauma.[1]

Subdural hemorrhages (SDH) and subarachnoid hemorrhages (SAH) can arise from either acceleration/deceleration forces or blunt impact, which injure "bridging" vessels that cross the subarachnoid and dura mater. The bridging veins penetrating the dura mater are very thin (10 µm) and do not have additional connective tissue support like the larger bridging veins within the subarachnoid space, which makes them more prone to injury.[1] This is why SDH occur at a higher frequency than SAH. Although traditionally called subdural hemorrhage, the blood is intradural in location within a cleavage plane in the outermost part of the dura mater, the dura border cell layer.

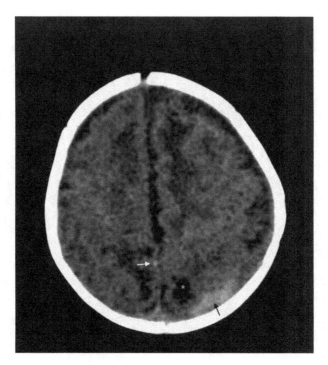

FIGURE 20.2. Unenhanced head CT showing hemorrhage in sulcus (white arrow) of right posteromedial parietal lobe. Partially hemorrhagic left frontoparietal convexity subdural hemorrhage (SDH) with layering hyperdense hemorrhage posteriorly (black arrow). Focal contusional cleft in left posteromedial parietal subcortical white matter near the gray–white junction appearing as a triangular cystic area (white*). Contusional clefts are highly characteristic and specific for abusive head trauma and are a distinct type of parenchymal laceration due to shearing injury in the very young (usually under 5 months of age), as shearing forces preferentially injure and tear the unmyelinated subcortical white matter at gray–white junction of gyral crests. They will have areas of hemorrhage in the cleft that can be well seen on susceptibility weighted MRI sequences but that may not be apparent on a head CT.

On a head CT, subdural collections can cross sutures and typically have concave margins. Bilateral subdural collections are common in the setting of abusive head trauma.[2,3] The vast majority of subdural collections due to abusive head injury are hemorrhagic in nature. However, acute simple subdural collections without hemorrhagic components, known as subdural effusions (also called post-traumatic subdural hygromas), can also occur acutely after trauma. Subdural hemorrhagic collections can present with a wide range of CT densities, and the appearance of SDH does not necessarily correlate to the timing of injury.

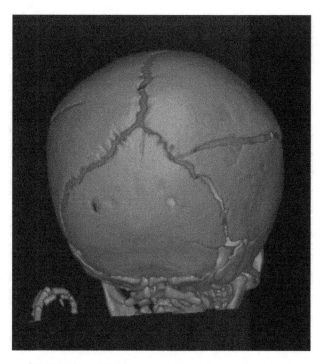

FIGURE 20.3. Shaded surface 3D reformats of the calvarium demonstrate bilateral noncommunicating parietal skull fractures, likely sequela of impact injury.

SAH are seen in the setting of both abusive and non-abusive head trauma and nontraumatic causes. On a head CT, SAH fill the sulcal spaces between parenchymal gyri or the basilar and suprasellar cisterns and conform to the outline of the space they occupy. It is important to distinguish subdural collections which denote pathology or trauma from prominent subarachnoid spaces, a benign finding in young infants. Vessels can be seen traversing the subarachnoid space collections but not subdural collections.[4]

Epidural hemorrhages (EDH) are collections of blood in the epidural space between the skull and dura mater, caused by damage to epidural arteries or veins arising from an impact injury, often with associated skull fractures. On head CT, EDH appear as a biconvex or lentiform collection (Figure 20.4) compared to the classic biconcave margins of the subdural collections, and are more likely to exert regional mass effect on the adjacent brain than a subdural collection of a similar size. Unlike subdural collections, EDH usually do not cross calvarial suture lines unless there is

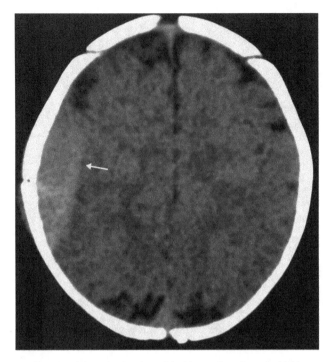

FIGURE 20.4. There is a right parietal region epidural hemorrhage (arrow) with biconvex margins noted adjacent to a right parietal bone fracture (*), which is not as well seen on this non-bone algorithm image.

a fracture crossing a suture or sutural diastasis. EDH can progress quickly, causing mass effect and herniation, especially if there is an arterial source of bleeding. Children can have the classic "lucid interval" prior to neurologic deterioration with an EDH, but this is not always present.

Interpretation of Head CT in Infants

Comprehensive evaluation of the head on CT involves assessing for ventricular size, mass effect and herniation, extra axial collections and hemorrhages, parenchymal masses and hemorrhages, preservation of gray–white differentiation in the brain parenchyma, evaluation of the scalp for hematoma, and complete evaluation of the skull for fractures, including at the skull base. See images Figure 20.5 a, 20.5b, 20.5c, 20.5d to review normal anatomy on a head CT including the 4th ventricle, 3rd ventricle, lateral ventricles, normal gray white differentiation and absence of extra axial fluid collections.

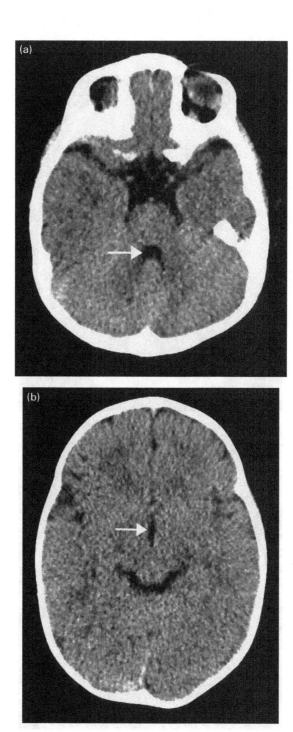

FIGURES 20.5a, 20.5b, 20.5c, 20.5d. Representative images at 4 different levels of a normal head CT in a 3-month-old. (a) At the level of the cerebellum. Note the normal size of the fourth ventricle (arrow) and the normal shape of the suprasellar cistern. (b) At the level of the thalamus and midbrain. Note the normal size of the third ventricle (arrow). (c) At the level of the body of lateral ventricles (star). (d) Above the level of the lateral ventricles. Note the normal appearance of the gray–white differentiation in an infant, absence of extra axial collections and mass effect.

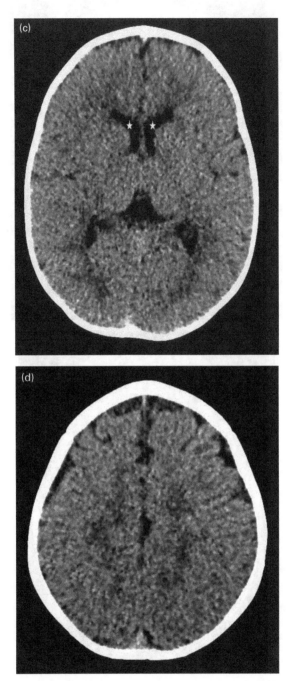

FIGURES 20.5a, 20.5b, 20.5c, 20.5d. Continued

PRESENTATION OF ABUSIVE HEAD TRAUMA

The acute presentation of abusive head trauma (AHT) is variable and can include irritability, lethargy, altered mental status, seizures, respiratory compromise, vomiting, fever, brief resolved unexplained event (BRUE), and poor feeding. While symptoms of a severe head trauma will present within hours of the time of injury, smaller intracranial injuries can have subtler or more ongoing symptoms.

Because the signs and symptoms of AHT can be subtle and mimic other common disease processes, approximately 30% are missed on the initial presentation.[5] An analysis of missed cases of AHT revealed viral gastroenteritis to be the most common erroneous diagnosis.[5] In other cases, symptoms were attributed to infections (otitis media, upper respiratory infection, sepsis, urinary tract infection, and meningitis) or were thought to be related to seizures, reflux, or benign increase in head circumference.

The physical examination of a child with AHT can be surprisingly unremarkable. Children with AHT may have no external signs of injury and may simply present with vomiting or fussiness; therefore, a high index of suspicion is important. Subtle, unexplained, or poorly explained injuries may be present on exam, such as bruising, oral injuries like a frenulum tear, or subconjunctival hemorrhages (the "red spot" in the eye of our patient). These are known as sentinel injuries and should raise concern for abuse in non-mobile children[6] (Box 20.1). Infants cannot self-inflict these injuries, and routine care should not cause those findings. Sentinel injuries themselves usually do not require treatment but are often associated with internal

---

BOX 20.1   **Sentinel Injuries**

Definition: Sentinel injuries are subtle, possibly abusive injuries in infants who are developmentally unable to cruise.

Bruising

Intra-oral injury
- Frenulum tear
- Palate bruising
- Tongue bruising

Subconjunctival hemorrhage not present at birth

Burns

---

injuries such as fractures, abdominal injuries, and ICH. Sentinel injuries may precede more severe or life-threatening injuries if abuse continues.

Common histories obtained in the setting of AHT are minor trauma, such as a short distance fall, or no history of trauma at all. While minor head injuries including skull fracture with or without associated *small* SDH, EDH, or SAH can sometimes be seen with short-distance falls (approximately 4 feet or less), this mechanism is unlikely to explain more extensive ICH, parenchymal contusion, or hypoxic-ischemic injury.[7,8] In cases when the veracity of a history is in question, discussion with a pediatric neuroradiologist and/or child abuse specialist can be helpful.

DIFFERENTIAL DIAGNOSIS

While commonly seen with abusive injury, ICH is not specific for abuse.[9] Birth-related SDH can be seen in the first month of life with both vaginal and cesarean deliveries but usually measure less than 3 mm, overlay the parieto-occipital lobes and tentorium, and self-resolve in the first 4 weeks of life.[2] High convexity interhemispheric or posterior fossa location SDH are significantly associated with abusive head injury in children over 1 month of age.[2,3]

Congenital bleeding disorders causing ICH, such as factor deficiencies, platelet abnormalities, or fibrinogen disorders, are exceedingly rare. Vitamin K deficiency can cause ICH and may be related to parental refusal of vitamin K at birth, maternal medications (i.e., anticonvulsants, anticoagulants), or fat malabsorption in the patient. Vitamin K deficiency appears prior to 8 months of age and is associated with an elevated prothrombin time (PT) and INR (international normalized ratio).

As described in a previous section, enlarged subarachnoid spaces can be seen on head CT in some infants, also named benign extra-axial fluid (BEAF) and benign enlarged subarachnoid spaces of infancy (BESSI). These infants usually have larger head circumferences on exam but are otherwise asymptomatic.

Glutaric aciduria type 1 (an inherited metabolic condition), scurvy, and Menkes disease can also present with ICH, although these would not be diagnoses made in the ED.

MEDICAL MANAGEMENT OF EXTRA-AXIAL HEMORRHAGE

Priority should be placed on emergent aspects of care such as airway, breathing, circulation, positioning, spinal precautions, normothermia, normocarbia, euglycemia, seizure control, mannitol or hypertonic saline, and neurosurgery involvement.[10] Please see Table 20.1 for further details on acute management of traumatic brain injury. Admission is the usual course of action, even if only for observation. Disposition to the regular floor or the intensive care unit (ICU) depends on clinical presentation, need for frequent neurologic checks, or close monitoring of labs. All children with epidural hemorrhages should receive pediatric neurosurgical consultation.

Neurosurgery consultation is valuable in cases of ICH, particularly in cases with complex neuroimaging results or when non-accidental trauma is a consideration. Discussion with a pediatric neuroradiologist can also help clarify details of difficult head CT results or need for further imaging.

MEDICAL EVALUATION FOR ABUSIVE HEAD TRAUMA

If there is concern for AHT, additional workup can be initiated in the ED and completed in the inpatient setting. If the patient is under 2 years old and is stable, obtain a skeletal survey.[11] It is reasonable to consider a skeletal survey in children over 2 years old if you think the patient cannot communicate pain from a bony injury (limited verbal communication, lack of sensation, unresponsive, or distracting injuries, etc.).[12,13] A skeletal survey differs from a babygram in that it includes 20 or more separate higher-quality images, which are necessary to identify subtle fractures. Obtaining AST (aspartate aminotransferase), ALT (alanine aminotransferase), and lipase values to screen for occult intra-abdominal injury is indicated for patients less than 5 years old with concern for abusive injuries.[14] If either the AST or ALT is ≥80 or if there is obvious abdominal trauma, including bruising, obtain a CT with IV contrast of the abdomen and pelvis.[14] MRI of the head and cervical spine are recommended in cases of ICH with concern for AHT, as MRI can further delineate injuries or identify non-abusive conditions.[2,11]

Consider obtaining blood prior to transfusion (if blood products are needed) to evaluate for a possible bleeding disorder, although rare. Basic

TABLE 20.1 **Emergency Treatment Strategies for Neurotrauma**

ATLS Primary Assessment	Airway: consider respiratory support or intubation if patient is not adequately oxygenating, ventilating, or protecting the airway. Breathing: assess for lung aeration or issues that could impede respiration (hemothorax, pneumothorax, rib fractures, etc.). Circulation: pulses and blood pressure. Keep in mind normal pediatric vital signs, the need to maintain cerebral perfusion pressure, and Cushing's triad (hypertension, bradycardia, respiratory changes). Disability: obtain a pediatric GCS and examine pupils. Exposure: completely undress the patient and examine for other injuries. Remember this can decrease body temperature.
Positioning	Consider spinal precautions and elevating the head of the bed to 30 degrees.
Ventilation	Target normocarbia (CO_2 of 35–40).
Temperature	Maintain normothermia. Prophylactic hypothermia has not been shown to be effective. Recheck temperatures frequently in the trauma bay.
Hyperosmolar therapy	Consider giving mannitol or 3% saline for ICP control (ex. poor or declining neurologic exam, hypertension, bradycardia). Consider agent availability, patient volume status, and serum sodium when choosing between mannitol and 3% saline.
Analgesics, sedatives, paralytics	Be mindful of drug effects on hemodynamics and neurologic examination.
Antiepileptics	Treat clinical seizures and consider seizure prophylaxis per your institutional protocol.
Imaging	Obtain non-contrast head CT to determine extent of injury and need for neurosurgical intervention.
Consult neurosurgery	To determine if OR craniotomy or ICP monitor placement is needed.
Corticosteroids	NOT recommended as a treatment for increased ICP.

laboratory testing in an AHT evaluation includes complete blood count (CBC), PT, partial thromboplastin time (PTT), INR, Factor VIII (8), d-dimer, fibrinogen, and if the patient is male, also Factor IX (9).[11]

A significant proportion of patients with abusive head trauma will have retinal hemorrhages, so ophthalmology consultation is indicated for abuse evaluations.[11] A dilated eye exam can be delayed until the patient is more stable if the pupillary response is necessary for neurologic monitoring.

MANDATED REPORTING

One of the most important considerations is a prompt report to Child Protective Services and/or law enforcement if child physical abuse is suspected. Also consider siblings or other children in the same care environment who might also be abused—they should also have a medical evaluation.[15]

KEY POINTS

- Abusive head trauma can have a subtle presentation, such as fussiness, vomiting, or a sentinel injury.
- A sentinel injury is an unexplained or poorly explained injury in a non-mobile child, such as a bruise, intra-oral injury, or subconjunctival hemorrhage not related to birth trauma that may precede more severe abusive injuries.
- In cases of suspected abuse in a young child, obtain labs and imaging (complete skeletal survey when appropriate) to evaluate for other injuries.
- Any injury where abuse is a possibility should be reported to Child Protective Services.
- Children in the same care environment also need medical evaluations for injuries.

- Carefully evaluate head CTs for subdural collections, which can vary in size and density and may be missed if small, isodense to CSF, and positioned along the vertex. Reviewing both coronal and sagittal plane images in addition to axial plane images can improve the detection of these collections.
- Do not confuse hypodense subdural effusions, which can indicate pathology, for benign enlargement of subarachnoid spaces seen in infancy (BESSI). If cortical vessels travel within the fluid collection, it is a subarachnoid collection, but an absence of crossing cortical vessels favors a subdural collection.
- Review 3D reformats of the calvarium alongside coronal and sagittal reformats in bone algorithm (the "bone window") to detect subtle nondisplaced skull fractures.
- If there are unexplained extra-axial collections on a head CT, a brain MRI can be done as an inpatient to better characterize these collections and detect possible additional injuries.

References

1. Wittschieber D, Karger B, Pfeiffer H, et al. Understanding subdural collections in pediatric abusive head trauma. *Am J Neuroradiol*. 2019;40:388–395.
2. Gunda D, Cornwell BO, Dahmoush HM, et al. Pediatric CNS imaging of NAT: beyond subdural hematomas. *Radiographics*. 2019;39:213–228.
3. Orman G, Kralik SF, Meoded A, et al. MRI findings in pediatric abusive head trauma: a review. *J Neuroimaging*. 2020;30:15–27.
4. Kuruvilla LC. Benign enlargement of sub-arachnoid spaces in infancy. *J Pediatr Neurosci*. 2014;9:129–131.
5. Jenny C, Hymel KP, Ritzen A, et al. Analysis of missed cases of abusive head trauma. *JAMA*. 1999;281:621–626.
6. Sheets LK, Leach ME, Koszewski IJ, et al. Sentinel injuries in infants evaluated for child physical abuse. *Pediatrics*. 2013;131:701–707.
7. Tung, GA. Imaging of abusive head trauma. In: Jenny C, ed., *Child Abuse and Neglect: Diagnosis, Treatment, and Evidence*. St. Louis, MO: Elsevier; 2011:373–390.
8. Hedlund, GL. Abusive head trauma: Extra-axial hemorrhage and nonhemic collections. In: Kleinman PK, ed., *Diagnostic Imaging of Child Abuse*. Cambridge: Cambridge University Press; 2015:394–452.

9. Greeley, CS. Conditions confused with head trauma. In: Jenny C, ed., *Child Abuse and Neglect: Diagnosis, Treatment, and Evidence*. St Louis, MO: Elsevier; 2011:441–450.

10. Kochanek, PM, Tasker RC, Carney N, et al. Guidelines for the management of pediatric severe traumatic brain injury, third edition: update of the Brain Trauma Foundation guidelines, executive summary. *Pediatr Crit Care Med*. 2019;20(3):280–289.

11. Christian CW, Crawford-Jakubiak JE, Flaherty EG, et al. The evaluation of suspected child physical abuse. *Pediatrics*. 2015;135(5):e1337–e1354.

12. Di Petro MA, Brody AS, Cassady CI, et al. Diagnostic imaging of child abuse, section on radiology. *Pediatrics* 2009;123(5):1430–1435.

13. Lindberg DM, Berger RP, Reynolds MS, et al. Yield of skeletal survey by age in children referred to abuse specialists. *J Pediatr*. 2014;164(4):1268–1273.

14. Lindberg DM, Makaroff K, Harper N, et al. Utility of hepatic transaminases to recognize abuse in children. *Pediatrics*. 2009;124(2):509–516.

15. Lindberg DM, Shapiro RA, Laskey AL, et al. Prevalence of abusive injuries in siblings and household contacts of physically abused children. *Pediatrics*. 2012;130(2): 193–201.

16. Choudhary AK, Servaes S, Slovis TL, et al. Consensus statement on abusive head trauma in infants and young children. *Pediatr Radiol*. 2018;48:1048–1065.

21 Ripping Apart My Heart

Thomas P. Conway, George C. Koberlein, and Francesca M. Bullaro

Case Study

A 15-year-old male was brought to a pediatric trauma center after being struck by a motor vehicle going approximately 50 mph. Witnesses stated that he was thrown over the vehicle on impact. On arrival at the Emergency Department (ED), he reports significant chest pain. He denies headache, neck pain, difficulty breathing, nausea, vomiting, or back pain. The patient denies any past medical history and reports no allergies. Vital signs include a pulse of 120 BPM, respiratory rate of 26 bpm, blood pressure of 146/76 mmHg, and oxygen saturation (SpO$_2$) of 100%. Primary survey includes an intact airway, unlabored breathing with bilateral breath sounds. Circulation is stable with pulses throughout. Glasgow Coma Scale (GCS) is 15 on arrival. Secondary survey is remarkable for a chest exam which includes intact clavicles, symmetrical chest rise without crepitus, and superficial abrasions noted to the left chest. Abdominal exam is soft with tenderness, guarding, and superficial abrasions over left hemiabdomen. The remainder of the exam is unremarkable.

What do I do now?

DISCUSSION

Evaluating for pediatric thoracic trauma includes the consideration of a multitude of pathologies, including pneumothorax, hemothorax, pulmonary contusion, pericardial tamponade, tracheobronchial injury, diaphragm rupture, myocardial contusion, rib fractures, flail chest, and, blunt thoracic vascular injury (Figures 21.1a–21.1c). Our patient presents with a high-impact mechanism of injury and obvious blunt chest trauma with complaints of chest pain. Given this presentation, a thoracic injury, including a vascular injury, needs to be strongly considered. Timely decision-making is imperative in diagnosing and guiding management of blunt thoracic trauma. The chest radiograph is the next step in management to better delineate pulmonary and vascular injury. A majority of chest trauma is secondary to blunt injury, with <15% representing penetrating trauma, with an overall mortality of 15%.[1] An organized approach to the pediatric trauma patient is centered in the principles of Advanced Trauma Life Support (ATLS), teaching a timely and systematic primary and secondary survey. Chest wall trauma should focus on the assessment of airway, breathing, circulation, disability, and exposure upon immediate arrival of the patient.

The approach to pediatric chest trauma differs from the treatment of adults in several anatomical aspects. First, the mediastinum of children is more mobile, making the possibility of tension pneumothorax, cardiac

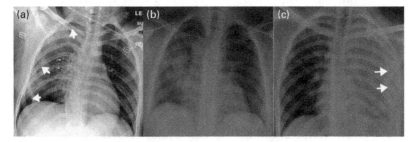

FIGURES 21.1a, 21.1b, AND 21.1c. Supine chest x-rays in three different patients with trauma from motor vehicle accidents. (a) Right-sided pneumothorax with a visceral pleural line (arrows) separating the aerated collapsing lung from the pleural air (devoid of lung markings). (b) Right lung contusion in the setting of trauma. (c) Large left pleural fluid from a traumatic hemothorax (arrows). Note the diffuse veiling opacification of the left hemithorax from layering of pleural fluid.

tamponade, and obstructive shock more likely. Rather than ossified adult structures, children's ribs are more cartilaginous, tending to absorb force in a bending fashion rather than fracturing, which may transmit force into the lungs or mediastinum.[1] In addition, pediatric resuscitation management is guided through a careful physical exam and awareness that pediatric patients compensate through an increase in heart rate to maintain cardiac output. The presence of hypotension is an ominous sign in the pediatric trauma resuscitation and should trigger a more aggressive resuscitation, and a search for the source of bleeding.

The primary survey of our patient would necessitate the stabilization of airway, breathing, and circulation. Careful inspection of the thorax for bilateral rise and fall of the chest, in addition to careful palpation for rib fractures (specifically rib 1 and 2), will guide assessment, although 30%–50% of patients will not show direct signs of trauma.[2] Trauma imaging of our patient would include an anteroposterior (AP) chest x-ray, AP pelvic radiograph, and adjunct imaging with focused assessment with sonography (FAST). Chest radiography is the primary imaging means in evaluating pediatric patients in the setting of blunt thoracic trauma. Etiologies such as rib fractures, pneumothorax, pulmonary contusions, as well as additional pulmonary and mediastinal pathologies, can be assessed by radiography, and often it is the only imaging modality that is required. Once the patient is stabilized, the decision to obtain further imaging must be considered.

During the primary survey of our patient, a screening trauma chest radiograph was obtained (Figure 21.2a), demonstrating an abnormal widened appearance of the mediastinum, which in the setting of trauma is concerning for vascular injury. The widening is apparent when compared to a normal patient of the same age (Figure 21.2b). If the patient is hemodynamically stable, this finding would prompt an emergent contrast enhanced computed tomography (CT) exam; specifically when vascular injury is suspected, a computed tomography angiography (CTA) is performed. The contrast needs to be injected at a higher speed with typically a larger bore IV and a power injector. The time between contrast administration and image acquisition is shorter than for a normal chest CT, so as to highlight the vasculature. Various articles advocate for the use of chest CTA in the setting of trauma when there is mediastinal widening, as vascular injury must

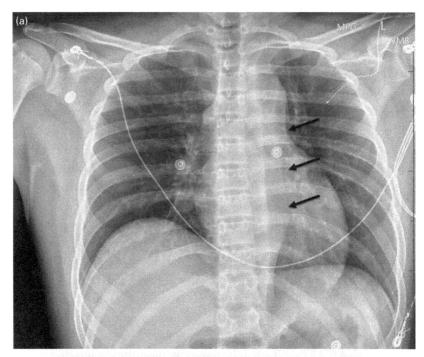

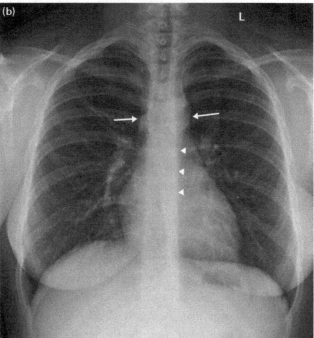

FIGURES 21.2a AND 21.2b. (a) Supine chest x-ray. This screening trauma radiograph of the chest demonstrates widening of the mediastinal and paraspinal soft tissues on the left (arrows). This appearance is concerning for an underlying vascular injury in the setting of blunt chest trauma and further imaging would be indicated. Note, the remainder of the radiograph is unremarkable. (b) Compare with a normal adolescent chest radiograph (different patient) with normal width of the superior mediastinum (arrows) and normal paraspinal soft tissues (arrowheads).

be excluded. Further, there is growing support that chest CTA should only be utilized when vascular injury is suspected.[3,4] Outside of vascular injury, chest CT does not yield significant change in acute trauma management and should only be performed in a patient that is deemed hemodynamically stable and not at risk for immediate decompensation. In our case scenario, a traumatic aortic pseudoaneurysm injury was discovered (Figures 21.3a, 21.3b, 21.4a, and 21.4b).

Traumatic aortic injury accounts for 2.1% of pediatric trauma deaths; however, this is rare, with incidence 0.1%–7.4% among children with blunt chest trauma.[2] Mechanisms of injury include motor vehicle collisions, motorcycle collisions, and falls.[5] Although over 85% of these patients die before reaching the hospital, early detection and intervention

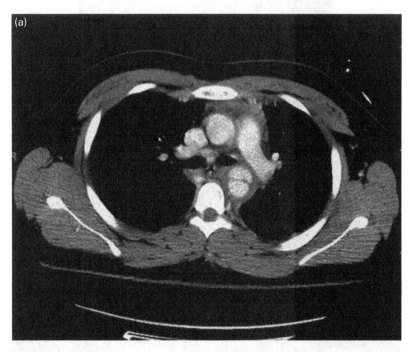

FIGURES 21.3a AND 21.3b. CT with contrast. (a) Axial image demonstrates a pseudoaneurysm, a contained rupture of the aorta, just distal to the aortic isthmus. (b) Sagittal image at the same level as (a), the pseudoaneurysm can be seen as a small outpouching along the lesser curvature of the aorta. These most commonly occur just distal to the aortic isthmus in the setting of trauma.

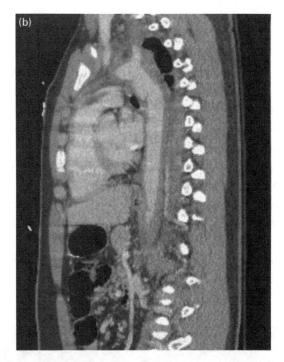

FIGURES 21.3a AND 21.3b. Continued

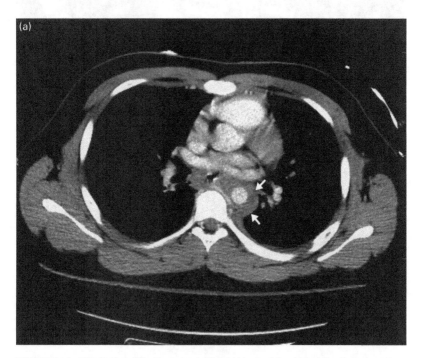

FIGURES 21.4a AND 21.4b. CT with contrast. (a) Axial image of the descending thoracic aorta demonstrating para-aortic hematoma (arrows), which accounts for the widened mediastinum and paraspinal soft tissues on the trauma x-ray. (b) Coronal image of the descending thoracic aorta demonstrates the hematoma along the length of the aorta (arrows), which one can better correlate with the initial x-ray.

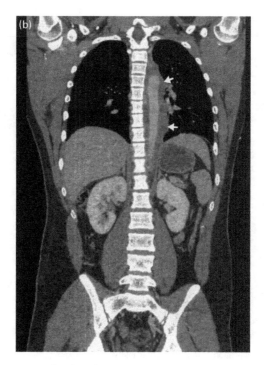

FIGURES 21.4a AND 21.4b. Continued

may improve morbidity and mortality.[6] Aortic injury occurs from the deceleration tearing force on the intimal walls, often causing a full thickness injury. The injuries occur at the site of aortic attachments and may form periaortic hematomas as well. These injuries may be seen on portable chest x-ray by the presence of mediastinal widening, indistinct aortic knob, left pleural effusion, thickening of the paratracheal stripe, or tracheal deviation. Chest CT scan, more specifically chest CTA, increases both sensitivity and specificity of blunt aortic injury, allowing visualization of aortic pseudoaneurysms, changes in aortic contour, thrombi, or contrast extravasation.[7] Once identified, aortic injury may be classified as follows (shown in Figure 21.5):[5]

- Grade I: Intimal tear
- Grade II: Intramural hematoma
- Grade III: Pseudoaneurysm
- Grade IV: Aortic rupture.

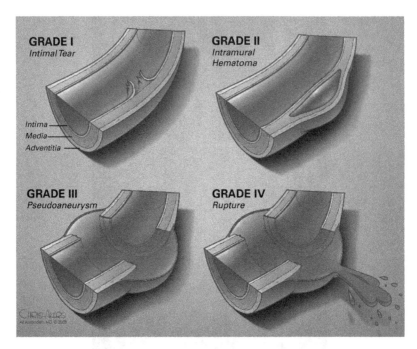

FIGURE 21.5. Classification of traumatic aortic injury.

Source: Reprinted from W. Anthony Lee, Jon S. Matsumura, R. Scott Mitchell, Mark A. Farber, Roy K. Greenberg, Ali Azizzadeh, Mohammad Hassan Murad, Ronald M. Fairman. Endovascular repair of traumatic thoracic aortic injury: clinical practice guidelines for the society of vascular surgery. *Journal of Vascular Surgery* 2011;53(1):187–192. Copyright 2011 with permission from Elsevier.

While grade I injuries may be treated conservatively with resuscitation and blood pressure management to avoid hypertension, grades II and beyond require operative repair. Current literature has identified a decrease in both morbidity and mortality by utilizing thoracic endovascular aortic repair (TEVAR) over the historical open thoracotomy, although pediatric data remain limited based on incidence.[8]

As illustrated by our case, blunt thoracic injury, specifically aortic injury, remains both a rare and challenging diagnosis to make. With prompt initiation of ATLS practices and rapid resuscitation, these patients may be identified with advanced imaging modalities, allowing for more timely treatment.

References

1. Haynes, J. *Pediatric Thoracic Trauma*. Children's Hospital of Richmond at VCU. October 10, 2015.
2. Pabon-Ramos W, et al. Radiologic evaluation of blunt thoracic aortic injury in pediatric patients. *Am J Roentgenol*. 2009;194:1197–1203.
3. Golden J, et al. Limiting chest computed tomography in the evaluation of pediatric thoracic trauma. *J Trauma Acute Care Surg*. 2016 Aug;81(2):271–277.
4. Holscher CM, et al. Chest computed tomography imaging for blunt pediatric trauma: not worth the radiation risk. *Journal of Surg Res*. 2013 Sep;184(1):352–357.
5. Trust M, Teixeria P. Blunt trauma of the aorta, current guidelines. *Cardiol Clin*. 2017;35:441–451.
6. Whizar-Lugo V, et al. Chest trauma: an overview. *J Anesth Crit Care*. 2015;3:1–11.
7. Kaewlai R, et al. Multidetector CT of blunt thoracic trauma. *RadioGraphics*. 2008;28:1555–1570.
8. Ramsuchit B, Cheatham M. Management of blunt thoracic aortic injury. *Surg Crit Care*. 2021:1–4.

22 The Unlucky Hit!

McKenzie Montana, Robert L. Gates, and Zachary Burroughs

Case Study

A 7-year-old previously healthy boy presents to the Emergency Department (ED) with abdominal pain. He was practicing his batting swing while his friend was up to bat. When his friend hit the ball, the bat flew out of his hand and hit the boy in the abdomen. He immediately felt pain but continued playing the game. His pain progressively worsened, and he had several episodes of nonbilious emesis throughout the rest of the day. Several hours later, his mom noticed a large bruise across his abdomen. Acetaminophen provided some relief. She brought him to the ED for further evaluation. Upon arrival, he was tachycardic to 117 BPM and normotensive at 98/70mmHg. He had moderate tenderness to palpation and a 10cm linear contusion on the left upper quadrant of his abdomen. His extremities were well perfused, and his capillary refill was 2 seconds. The remainder of the exam was normal.

What do you do now?

INTRODUCTION

The approach to pediatric trauma begins with the primary survey and then proceeds to the secondary survey. Carefully conduct a primary survey to evaluate the airway, breathing, circulation, disability, and neurologic status, and completely expose every patient presenting to the ED following a traumatic event. Traumatic abdominal injuries may be subtle, and vital signs are essential considerations in the initial evaluation. Tachycardia is an early abnormality in children suffering from intra-abdominal bleeding. Additionally, pallor or prolonged capillary refill are signs of poor perfusion and may indicate hemodynamic instability. Children can lose up to 30% of their blood volume (class III shock) before manifesting any significant change in blood pressure. Hypotension is a late finding. Therefore, it is important for providers not to be misled by a compensated blood pressure in the setting of presumed abdominal hemorrhage.

The secondary survey is a head-to-toe assessment to identify any other significant injuries. Unlike other traumatic injuries, blunt abdominal trauma may not present with obvious physical exam findings. The mechanism of injury and a focused history should guide the physical exam and further diagnostic workup. In the above scenario, there is a clear mechanism leading to the patient's abdominal pain. Physical exam findings that are associated with abdominal organ injuries include abdominal tenderness, ecchymoses, seatbelt sign, distension, rigidity, rebound, or guarding. The patient may also complain of shoulder pain, which may be a referred pain from irritation of the diaphragm via the phrenic nerve. Especially in younger children, the diagnosis can be difficult due to vague complaints and nonspecific exam findings.

Multiple organs are at risk in the pediatric abdominal trauma patient. Specifically, the spleen and liver are the most commonly injured organs. These organs are poorly protected by a child's smaller, more compliant rib cage, as well as decreased abdominal fat and muscle mass. Additionally, these organs take up more surface area relative to a child's smaller body. Splenic and hepatic injuries may be contained within the organ, or can cause brisk bleeds into the abdominal cavity that may, otherwise, present with subtle findings on physical exam. Additionally, injury to the bowel and mesentery are often subtle, frequently are not diagnosed with imaging, and may have a delayed presentation of days to weeks.

Therefore, the initial assessment of the child should focus on hemodynamic stability vs. instability. This differentiation will drive the diagnostic evaluation and management, which is drastically different between the two.

THE UNSTABLE PATIENT

The unstable pediatric abdominal trauma patient shows signs of hemorrhagic shock. The hemodynamically unstable pediatric trauma patient will have tachycardia (if in extremis the patient may have bradycardia). The patient will have weak distal pulses and prolonged capillary refill, in addition to cool and pale extremities. Peripheral vasoconstriction causes a "cold shock" presentation. As mentioned previously, hypotension is a late finding.[1]

Resuscitation should be initiated immediately in patients with evidence of hemodynamic instability. Pediatric blood volume varies by age group (90–100mL/kg: premature infant; 80–90mL/kg: term infant to 3 months; 70 mL/kg: >3 months). All active, visible bleeding should be stopped with direct pressure. Extremity bleeding that cannot be controlled with direct pressure may require a tourniquet application. The emergency medicine physician should initiate resuscitation with a 20 mL/kg bolus of crystalloid fluid. Likewise, it is crucial to establish a baseline hemoglobin and hematocrit (H&H), in addition to a type and screen. Of note, a patient's initial hematocrit may be normal in the setting of hemorrhage. The Shock Index Pediatric Age adjusted (SIPA, Figure 22.1) should be calculated, and if elevated indicates a need for blood transfusion.[2] Additional crystalloid administration has been shown to increase mortality.[3] In addition, it has been shown that hemodilution due to excessive fluid causes increased transfusion requirements, prolonged prothrombin time (PT), and leads to multiorgan system failure. Massive transfusion is activated when a patient is in class IV hemorrhagic shock, which is defined as greater than 40% blood loss, receives 40ml/kg or 4 units of blood in 2 hours, undergoes complete blood volume replacement in 24 hours (approximately 1 unit in a 5 kg patient, 2 units in a 10 kg patient, or 4 units in greater than a 30 kg patient), and/or has the presence of life-threatening hemorrhage unlikely to

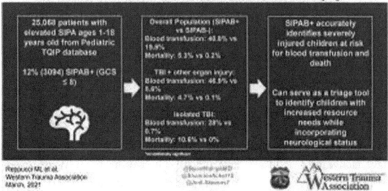

Pediatric Age-Adjusted Shock Index (SIPA) as a Tool for Predicting Outcomes in Children With or Without Traumatic Brain Injury

FIGURE 22.1.   Pediatric Age-Adjusted Shock Index (SIPA).

respond to fluids. Initially, blood products should be transfused in a 1:1 ratio of packed red blood cells (PRBCs) to fresh frozen plasma (FFP) and a directed pediatric massive transfusion protocol should be followed. Trauma induced coagulopathy occurs in 29%–57% of severely injured patients and is an independent predictor of mortality. Therefore, if available a viscoelastic hemostatic assay such as thromboelastography (TEG) or rotational thromboelastometry (ROTEM) should be drawn early to guide blood product administration.[4] The use of tranexamic acid (TXA) is promising, but not well studied in pediatrics.[5] All patients requiring greater than a 20 mL/kg of crystalloid resuscitation need to be at a pediatric trauma center for evaluation by a pediatric surgeon for determination of the need for operative intervention.

Extended focused assessment with sonography for trauma exam (e-FAST) is frequently used in pediatric trauma because it rapidly evaluates a patient and is not associated with radiation exposure. Unlike imaging with a CT, a FAST exam is performed in the trauma bay. It is a quick way for physicians to see blood in the pericardial sac or in the peritoneal cavity during the secondary survey. In pediatric patients the sensitivity of the exam is low, so physical exam, SIPA score, and response to fluid and blood product administration are important determinants for laparotomy.

Long et al. demonstrated in a large series of children that a positive FAST exam improves the ability to predict the need for early surgical intervention and that the accuracy is greater for detecting free fluid in hemodynamically unstable patients 2 hours after arrival in the ED. Abdominal CT scan in a hemodynamically unstable patient should be avoided because of potential for severe decompensation during the scan, while away from the trauma bay or operating room.[12]

THE STABLE PATIENT

Two categories of stable patients exist: patients with a normal mental status and signs and symptoms of abdominal trauma, and patients with an altered mental status and potential abdominal trauma. The stable pediatric abdominal trauma patient does not show signs of hemorrhagic shock.

For patients with an altered mental status (or intubated) and potential abdominal trauma, intracranial processes must be considered and appropriate imaging obtained. Patients with a normal mental status and abdominal trauma should be selectively imaged based on clinical findings. A study in 2013 looked at the use of CT scans in pediatrics and the estimated cancer risk. The authors suggested that the 4 million pediatric CT scans of the head, abdomen/pelvis, chest, or spine performed nationally each year are projected to cause 4,870 future cancers.[2] Therefore, the use of a CT scan should be intended for those that have clinically significant injuries to the abdominal organs where understanding the extent of the injury would change the management. To limit the exposure to radiation, Pediatric Emergency Care Applied Research Network (PECARN) created a prediction rule to determine children at a very low risk for intra-abdominal injury. The prediction rule consisted of (in descending order of importance) no evidence of abdominal wall trauma or seatbelt sign, Glasgow Coma Scale score greater than 13, no abdominal tenderness, no evidence of thoracic wall trauma, no complaints of abdominal pain, no decreased breath sounds, and no vomiting.[4] This study had a 97% sensitivity in ruling out the need for a pediatric patient to receive a CT scan. The prediction rule provided excellent external validation in a follow-up study.[5] Overall, if a patient meets the criteria, a CT scan should not be obtained.

Obtaining and trending the H&H, liver enzymes, and urinalysis can be helpful to indicate ongoing bleeding or an inflammatory process prior to obtaining a CT scan. In particular, an AST >120 IU/L and/or ALT >90 IU/L has been shown to be associated with liver injury.[13] A low hemoglobin, elevated liver enzymes, and hematuria warrant imaging with a CT to evaluate the extent of the organ injury and thus direct further therapy.

Sola et al. found that a negative FAST examination combined with normal liver enzymes was an effective screening tool for excluding an intra-abdominal injury, potentially eliminating the need for additional imaging. However, a systematic review and meta-analysis of prospective studies of point-of-care ultrasound FAST examinations found that the FAST examination cannot be used in isolation to exclude an intra-abdominal injury in children. Review of recent data also suggests that a hemodynamically stable child with a positive FAST examination should have a CT scan performed. About one-third of children do not develop free detectable intraperitoneal fluid with an intra-abdominal injury, contributing to the significantly high false-negative rate for US in some studies.

Following the CT scan, the injury patterns can be graded. The American Association for the Surgery of Trauma injury grading system for injuries to the spleen and liver are listed in Table 22.1. Essentially, the grade of injury depends on involvement of the subcapsular region extending to the vascular system. The more involvement of the organ, the higher the grade. More than one grade may be present in a trauma, but the highest grade will help direct the management (Figures 22.2–22.5).

On a contrast enhanced CT of the abdomen done for trauma, all solid organs should be checked for size, smooth contour, lack of space occupying lesions, presence of expected vascular pattern, and phase of enhancement. Figures 22.6a–22.6c exemplify a normal abdominal CT through the upper abdominal viscera, with labeling of critical structures.

The treatment of a stable patient with a bleeding abdominal organ entails volume resuscitation and controlling the pain. While in the ED, the patient must be made nothing by mouth (NPO) and started on maintenance intravenous fluids. Diet should be held in case the patient develops worsening bleeding that would require further intervention under a general

TABLE 22.1 **The American Association for the Surgery of Trauma Injury Scoring Scale**

Grade	Spleen	Liver
I	Subcapsular hematoma: <10% surface area Parenchymal laceration <1cm depth Capsular tear	Subcapsular hematoma <10% surface area Parenchymal laceration <1cm depth
II	Subcapsular hematoma: 10%–50% surface area Intraparenchymal hematoma <5 cm Parenchymal laceration 1–3 cm	Subcapsular hematoma 10%–50% surface area Intraparenchymal hematoma <10cm in diameter Laceration 1–3 cm in depth and <10cm length
III	Subcapsular hematoma >50% surface area Ruptured subcapsular or intraparenchymal hematoma >5cm	Subcapsular hematoma >50% surface area Ruptured subcapsular or parenchymal hematoma Intraparenchymal hematoma >10 cm Laceration >3cm depth Any injury in the presence of a liver vascular injury or active bleeding contained within liver parenchyma
IV	Any injury in the presence of a splenic vascular injury or active bleeding confined within splenic capsule Parenchymal laceration involving segmental or hilar vessels producing >25% devascularization	Parenchymal disruption involving 25%–75% of a hepatic lobe Active bleeding extending beyond the liver parenchyma into the peritoneum
V	Any injury in the presence of a splenic vascular injury with active bleeding extended beyond the spleen into the peritoneum Shattered spleen	Parenchymal disruption >75% of hepatic lobe Juxtahepatic venous injury to include retrohepatic vena cava and central major hepatic veins

The American Association for the Surgery of Trauma injury scoring scale updated in 2018. This grading system is the most widely used by radiologists. The grade of injury determines the management of blunt abdominal injuries.

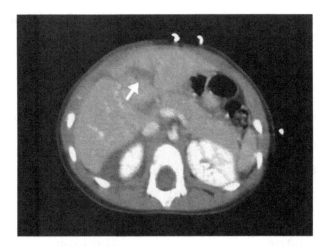

FIGURE 22.2. Grade III liver laceration. Axial contrast enhanced CT of the abdomen demonstrates a liver laceration (arrow) spanning more than 3cm into the parenchyma (liver surface extension not shown on this image).

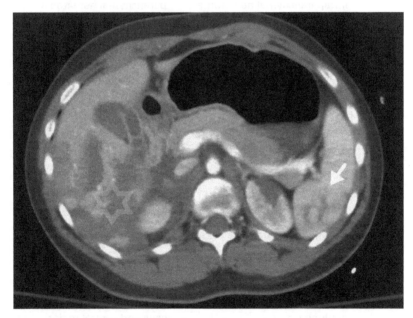

FIGURE 22.3. Grade V liver laceration with a grade II splenic laceration. Axial contrast enhanced CT of the abdomen demonstrates extensive liver parenchymal disruption (star) involving most of the right lobe. Also note splenic parenchymal lacerations measuring less than 3cm (arrow).

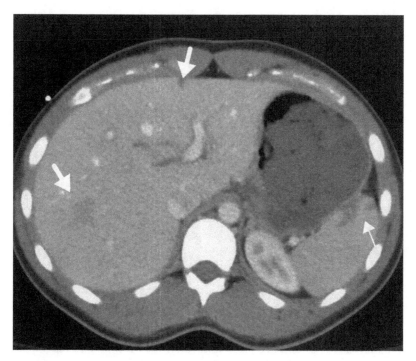

FIGURE 22.4. Grade II liver laceration with a grade I splenic laceration. Axial contrast enhanced CT of the abdomen demonstrates two liver lacerations (thick arrows) and a splenic laceration (thin arrow).

anesthetic. Pain management starts with 15 mg/kg of acetaminophen every 6 hours, and if unable to achieve adequate analgesia, then 0.05 mg/kg morphine every 2–4 hours may be added.

Grade of injury, in addition to hemodynamic stability, will assist in determining the disposition of the child.[14] If there is no evidence of solid organ laceration or hematoma, the child may be discharged home with instructions to return to the ED if they develop signs of solid organ injury, including syncope, pallor, significant abdominal pain, or emesis.

Children with grade I to III injuries may be admitted for a 24-hour observation period with monitoring of vital signs every 2–4 hours to identify transient hemodynamic instability. Diet can be started 8–12 hours after admission if they remain stable. Solid organ injuries grade IV and above

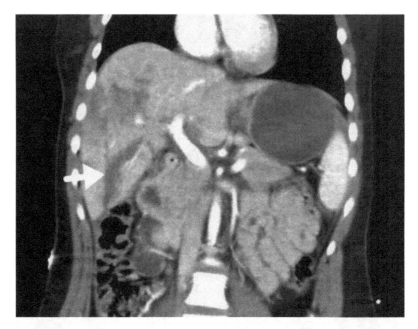

FIGURE 22.5.   Grade V liver laceration. Coronal section through a contrast enhanced abdominal CT demonstrates the severe parenchymal disruption of the right lobe of liver with deep lacerations (arrow) and intraparenchymal hematomas.

will need continuous hemodynamic monitoring in a pediatric intensive care unit (PICU) or step-down unit. They are discharged based upon clinical progress, usually in 24–48 hours (about 2 days). Following discharge, normal activity will need to be restricted for at least 3 weeks, and contact sports will need to be restricted for at least 6 weeks.

CASE CONCLUSION

The patient in the case scenario had evidence of abdominal trauma, endorsed abdominal pain, and had several episodes of vomiting. His clinical picture suggested evidence of intra-abdominal organ injury. A CT with contrast was obtained, revealing a grade III injury of his spleen. He was admitted to trauma service for pain control and maintenance fluids for 3 days. It was recommended to not return to baseball for approximately 6 weeks.

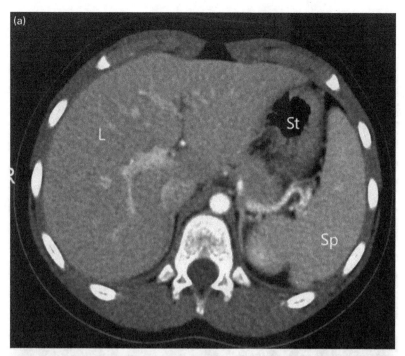

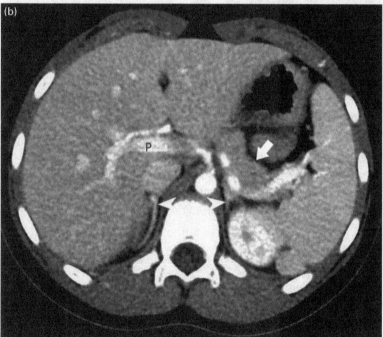

FIGURES 22.6a, 22.6b, AND 22.6c. Contrast enhanced CT in a 7-year-old with trauma. Sequential axial images through the upper abdomen in the soft tissue window. (a) Note normal enhancement of the liver (L), and spleen (Sp). Portal vein branching is seen within the liver. Stomach lies in the left upper quadrant (St). (b) Image at the level of the pancreas body and tail (white arrow). Normal portal vein (P) with the hepatic artery anterior to it is seen. Note the normal appearance of the adrenal glands (arrowheads). (c) Image at the level of the gallbladder demonstrates a distended gallbladder (arrow). Note the normal symmetric corticomedullary phase of renal enhancement. Bowel loops in the abdomen (star) are decompressed.

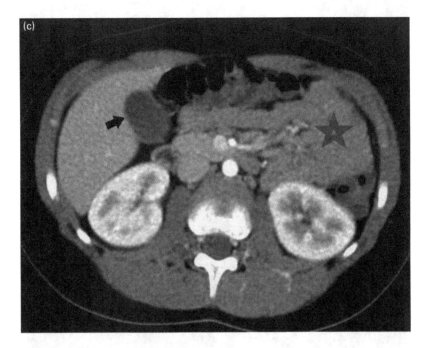

FIGURES 22.6a, 22.6b, AND 22.6c. Continued

KEY POINTS

- Tachycardia is the first change in vital signs of a child with hemorrhage.
- The abdominal organs are not well protected because of their compliant ribcage and poor abdominal musculature.
- Consider blood transfusion after a single 20 mg/kg bolus in a child with persistent tachycardia and poor perfusion.

TIPS FROM THE RADIOLOGIST

- e-FAST examination cannot be used in isolation to exclude an intra-abdominal injury in children, as one-third of children with intra-abdominal injury do not develop free detectable intraperitoneal fluid.

- PECARN criteria can be used to rule out the need for abdominal CT in the setting of trauma.
- The American Association for the Surgery of Trauma Injury Scoring Scale (AAST) staging of liver and splenic trauma aids in monitoring patients and guiding treatment.

Further Reading

1. Guralnick, S. Blunt abdominal trauma. *Pediatr Rev.* 2008;29(8):294–295.
2. Hobson M, Chima, R. Pediatric hypovolemic shock. *Open Pediatr Med J.* 2013;7(Suppl 1: M3):10–15.
3. Patel N, Alarcon, L. Blunt splenic trauma. *Am Assoc Surg Trauma.* 2012.
4. Holmes JF. Identifying Children at Very Low Risk of Clinically Important Blunt Abdominal Injuries. *Ann Emerg Med.* 2013 Aug;62(2);107–116.e2.
5. Fox S. Low risk for intra abdominal truama. *Pediatric EM Morsel.* January 2015. Pedemmorsels.com
6. Kozar RA, Crandall M, Shanmuganathan K, et al. Organ injury scaling 2018 update: spleen, liver, and kidney. *J Trauma Acute Care Surg.* 2018;85:1119–1122.
7. Springer E, Frazier SB, Arnold DH, Vukovic AA. External validation of a clinical prediction rule for very low risk pediatric blunt abdominal trauma. *Am J Emerg Med.* 2019 Sep;37(9):1643–1648. doi: 10.1016/j.ajem.2018.11.031. Epub 2018 Nov 23. PMID: 30502218.
8. Hussmann B, Lefering R, Kauther MD, Ruchholtz S, Moldzio P, Lendemans S; TraumaRegister DGU®. Influence of prehospital volume replacement on outcome in polytraumatized children. *Crit Care.* 2012 Oct 18;16(5):R201. doi: 10.1186/cc11809. PMID: 23078792; PMCID: PMC3682303.
9. Scaife ER, Rollins MD, Barnhart DC, Downey EC, Black RE, Meyers RL, Stevens MH, Gordon S, Prince JS, Battaglia D, Fenton SJ, Plumb J, Metzger RR. The role of focused abdominal sonography for trauma (FAST) in pediatric trauma evaluation. *J Pediatr Surg.* 2013 Jun;48(6):1377–83. doi: 10.1016/j.jpedsurg.2013.03.038. PMID: 23845633.

References

1. Hobson M, Chima, R. Pediatric hypovolemic shock. *Open Pediatr Med J.* 2013;7(Suppl 1: M3):10–15.
2. Phillips R, Meier M, Shahi N, Acker S, Reppicci M, Shirek G, Recicar J, Moulton S, Bensard D. Elevated pediatric age-adjued shock-index (SIP) in blunt solid organ injuries. *J Pediatr Surg.* 2021;56:401–404.

3. Polites SF, et al. Timing and volume of crystalloid and blood products in pediatric trauma: an Eastern Association of the Surgery of Trauma multicenter prospective observational study. *J Trauma Acute Care Surg*. 2020;89(1):36–42.

4. Cunningham AJ, Condron M, Schreiber MA, Azarow K, Hamiliton NA, Downie K, Long WB, Mawell BG, Jafri MA. Rotational thromboelastometry predicts transfusion and disability in pediatric trauma. *J Trauma Acute Care Surg*. 2019;88(1):134–140.

5. Beno S, Ackery AD, Callum J, Rizolli S. Traneximic acid in children: why not? *Crit Care*. 2014;18:313.

6. Miglioretti DL, Johnson E, Williams A, Greenlee RT, Weinmann S, Solberg LI, Feigelson HS, Roblin D, Flynn MJ, Vanneman N, Smith-Bindman R. The use of computed tomography in pediatrics and the associated radiation exposure and estimated cancer risk. *JAMA Pediatr*. 2013 Aug 1;167(8):700–707. doi: 10.1001/jamapediatrics.2013.311. PMID: 23754213; PMCID: PMC3936795.

7. Butts, C. Not So FAST: should this exam be used in children? *Emerg Med News*. Aug 2016.

8. Holmes JF, Lillis K, Monroe D, Borgialli D, Kerrey BT, Mahajan P, Adelgais K, Ellison AM, Yen K, Atabaki S, Menaker J, Bonsu B, Quayle KS, Garcia M, Rogers A, Blumberg S, Lee L, Tunik M, Kooistra J, Kwok M, Cook LJ, Dean JM, Sokolove PE, Wisner DH, Ehrlich P, Cooper A, Dayan PS, Wootton-Gorges S, Kuppermann N; Pediatric Emergency Care Applied Research Network (PECARN). Identifying children at very low risk of clinically important blunt abdominal injuries. *Ann Emerg Med*. 2013 Aug;62(2):107–116.e2. doi: 10.1016/j.annemergmed.2012.11.009. Epub 2013 Feb 1. PMID: 23375510.

9. Springer E, Frazier SB, Arnold DH, Vukovic AA. External validation of a clinical prediction rule for very low risk pediatric blunt abdominal trauma. *Am J Emerg Med*. 2019 Sep;37(9):1643–1648. doi: 10.1016/j.ajem.2018.11.031. Epub 2018 Nov 23. PMID: 30502218.

10. Kozar RA, Crandall M, Shanmuganathan K, et al. Organ injury scaling 2018 update: spleen, liver, and kidney. *J Trauma Acute Care Surg*. 2018;85:1119–1122.

11. Retzlaff T, Hirsch W, Till H, Rolle U. Is sonography reliable for the diagnosis of pediatric blunt abdominal trauma? *J Pediatr Surg*. 2010 May;45(5):912–915. doi: 10.1016/j.jpedsurg.2010.02.020. PMID: 20438925.

12. Long MK, Vohra MK, Bonnette A, Vega-Parra PD, Miller SK, Ayub E, WAng HE, Cardenas-Turanzas M, Gordon R, Ugalde IT, Allkian M, Smith HE. Focused assessment with sonography for trauma in predicting early surgical intervention in hemodynamically unstable children with blunt abdominal trauma. *J Am Coll Emerg Physicians Open*. 2022 Jan 27;3(1):e12650. PMID 35128532.

13. Zeeshan M, Hamidi M, O'Keefe T, Hanna K, Kulvatunyou N, Tang A, Joseph B. Pediatric liver injury: physical examination, FAST and serum transaminases can serve as a guide. *J Surg Res*. 2019 Oct;242:151–156. PMID: 31078899.

14. Gates RL, Price M, Cameron DB, Somme S, Ricca R, Oyetunji TA, Guner YS, Gosain A, Baird R, Lal DR, Jancelewicz T, Shelton J, Diefenbach KA, Grabowski J, Kawaguchi A, Dasgupta R, Downard C, Goldin A, Petty JK, Stylianos S, Williams R. Non-operative management of solid organ injuries in children: an American Pediatric Surgical Association Outcomes and Evidence Based Practice Committee systematic review. *J Pediatr Surg*. 2019 Aug;54(8):1519–1526. PMID: 30773395.

Index